The Fourth Wave: Digital Health
A New Era of Human Progress

By Paul Sonnier

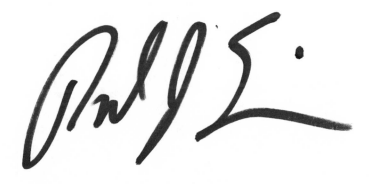

Stay abreast of the latest news relevant to The Fourth
Wave: Digital Health by subscribing to Paul Sonnier's
newsletter at FourthWaveBook.com or
StoryofDigitalHealth.com

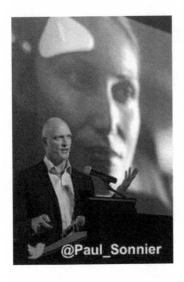

Point your iPhone or Android
smartphone camera at the QR
code and receive a prompt to
visit my website

Follow Paul on Twitter @Paul_Sonnier

Note: In this print version all references indicated by
underlined hyperlinked text can be accessed via the
digital Kindle version.

Copyright Notice

Dedication

To Ed Cahill and Brian Post, whose mentorship means the world to me. To Kim Whittemore, my trusted friend and advisor. And to my parents—Joe and Eva—for encouraging me to follow my bliss.

Table of Contents

Introduction 1

Definition...8

   Genomics 9

Cambrian Explosion 17

   Devices and Sensors..................................18

   Apps and Social Media 21

Key Factors 30

   Economics and Access..............................30

   Investing and Innovation Acceleration....................38

   Regulation 40

   Markets 47

Strategies...**50**

   Enhancement 56

   Multifaceted..61

   Adjacent 68

   Disruption...71

   Healthcare 73

      Telehealth...78

Opportunities **82**

   Chronic Disease..82

   Genetic Testing 88

Genome Sequencing 92

Gene Editing 93

Gene Therapy 96

Liquid Biopsies 99

Imaging 100

Autonomous Vehicles 103

Human Augmentation 104

Pandemics and Health Testing 109

Food Security 116

The Fourth Wave 122

Timeline 127

5G 129

Virtual Reality 131

Genomics 132

Inflection Point 134

Businesses and Organizations 134

People 136

Ride the Wave 136

Introduction

In 1989, shortly after enlisting in the U.S. Navy, I had my first experience working in digital health. Following basic training (aka boot camp) I entered my 'A' school to learn the fundamentals of electronics and digital computing in preparation for my job as an aviation electronics (avionics) technician. While I didn't foresee it at the time, this training—and other professional roles over the following two decades—would form the basis for my passion for digital health, ultimately leading to this book.

In the Navy, I diagnosed and repaired radio communications and navigation equipment used in military aircraft, including the F-14 Tomcat fighter jet and the EA-6B Prowler tactical signal-jamming aircraft. The avionics systems were vital to both aircraft navigation and the health and safety of the pilots, as were the emergency survival radios, which all pilots carried in their flight suits. The ejection seats in the aircraft, as well, were equipped with a survival kit containing an emergency radio beacon. In the event of an ejection from the aircraft, the beacon would automatically turn on and transmit a signal on the military air distress frequency (243 MHz), enabling search and rescue personnel to find the pilot and crew. The beacon could also be set for manual activation, which was useful if the aircraft went down in enemy held territory, where it wouldn't be desirable to immediately notify the enemy of the crew's location. Both the survival radio and emergency beacon are life-saving systems comprised of digital computing components. In other words, they are 'digital health'.

Following the Navy, I completed my bachelor's degree in manufacturing engineering technology and went to work in Seattle, WA for Boeing as a process improvement engineer in the electrical systems manufacturing center. A couple of years later, I took a role as a program coordinator in the avionics systems design team working on Boeing's 787 Dreamliner airplane program.

After six years at Boeing—and the completion of a master's degree in business administration (MBA)—I was struck by professional wanderlust and a desire to advance my career along a different path. This led me to change industries entirely, moving out of commercial aerospace and into the medical device field. I took a role at a startup, Calypso Medical Technologies (subsequently acquired by Varian Medical Systems), where I coordinated hardware and software design teams developing a novel medical device system. Marketed as 'GPS for the body', the system uses tiny beacon transponders—implanted into the prostate gland—that emit radio signals for use in focusing radiation beams used in cancer treatment. Benefits of the system include improved accuracy, enabling higher radiation doses and fewer treatments, as well as reduced risk of harming healthy surrounding tissues.

In 2008, I took a management role in San Diego, CA with cell phone-maker Motorola. While this was exciting in terms of career advancement and moving back to my hometown, the timing couldn't have been worse. Just one year prior, Apple had launched its first-generation iPhone and Motorola, caught off guard without a smartphone of their own, was in serious trouble. During my tenure at Motorola, however, I had volunteered at a professional organization named CommNexus San Diego (since renamed to EvoNexus and transformed into a startup incubator). It was there, while serving as a co-chair of the organization's Healthcare Communications Special Interest Group (SIG), that I was brought back to my roots in digital health. When I was impacted by Motorola's workforce downsizing in 2009, I threw myself into my co-chair role, learning as much as I could about the convergence of health, healthcare, and wireless technologies.

One of my CommNexus co-chairs was Donald Jones, who at that time was working for Qualcomm, the multinational semiconductor and wireless telecommunications equipment company. Intrigued by Jones' work evangelizing what he described as 'wireless health', I Googled his name and came across a YouTube video, in which he spoke about the many ways that wireless devices and communications are helping to improve health and healthcare. His comments about the size of the business markets also intrigued me.

Inspired and energized, I decided to share what I was learning with the world. Since I was active on the social networking website LinkedIn, I created a group named 'Wireless Health San Diego' and began sharing news and alerting members to upcoming professional events. At that time, there weren't nearly as many stories on the topic of digital health compared to what we see, but I noticed a few interesting trends. For one, people from around the globe were joining my 'little' group. News, as well, was occurring everywhere, and increasing in volume. The group was becoming a hub for discussing news and connecting professionals. In response, I decided to expand the geographic scope beyond San Diego and renamed the group to 'Wireless Health'.

Also at that time I encountered many terms to describe the emerging technology-based trends in health and healthcare. This lexicon included terms like telehealth and telemedicine, wireless health, mHealth (mobile health), health IT (aka health information technology), big data (when applied to health), genomics and genetics, personalized and precision medicine, digital health (though rarely used at the time), and of course the generic 'health tech'.

Concise terminology facilitates clear communication, as I knew from my experience overseeing and coordinating the work of cross-functional, interdisciplinary product development teams. In fact, it's a critical element to the success of researching, designing, developing, and manufacturing high tech systems. As such, from a communications standpoint, the plethora of terms bothered me. I felt this situation slowed progress and restrained the benefits that could be obtained. While I couldn't put my finger on it, there seemed to be something missing— something tying it all together.

Several years passed and a suitable, overarching term seemingly failed to appear. To my dismay, conversations around 'health tech' were a disarray of artificially partitioning terms, which helped reinforce the status quo rather than catalyze disruptive innovation.

The tectonic changes I was seeing had no name. No matter where I looked, I failed to find a common denominator for all of them much less a concise and suitable description for the revolutionary changes that appeared to be taking place.

This frustrating situation finally changed in December 2011, when Eric Topol, MD—whom I had met during my role as vice president at an industry organization called the Wireless-Life Sciences Alliance—published his book 'The Creative Destruction of Medicine: How the Digital Revolution Will Create Better Health Care'.

In reading Topol's book, I discerned two vital pieces of contextual information. First, Topol explicitly identified the Digital Revolution in the book's title and he described the many ways it was already changing and would continue to improve medicine and healthcare. Second, he included a chapter on genomics and pointed out the fundamental role of "chips and automated robotic systems" in accelerating genomics, particularly in medicine.

While thinking about the link between digital technology and genomics, I had an epiphany. Since 'digital' was clearly the common denominator for the myriad of health tech terms, the one I sought—though rarely used—was already in existence: digital health. Moreover, I saw that genomics rightfully belonged within the scope of digital health. The reasons for this—as I go into—extend beyond the acceleration of genomics by the Digital Revolution.

In early 2012, I renamed my LinkedIn group to Digital Health. Out of over one million groups on the platform at the time, this unique name was available, further indication that its significance was being missed. I also began promulgating my definition of digital health, articulating that it is the convergence of both the Digital Revolution and genomics with health, healthcare, living, and society. I became much more active on Twitter—now using the hashtag #DigitalHealth—which went viral.

My message began to resonate, and my group continued to grow, as did my influence. I soon found myself being contacted by organizations working to foster and accelerate digital health innovation, including the XPRIZE, where I served as a judge for a $2.5 million prize focused on the development of sensors for health and medical applications. I also worked with the World Economic Forum (WEF), which invited me to serve as a member of their Digital Health Global Agenda Council. In 2015, I had the honor of delivering my first keynote presentation at a conference in Seoul, Korea, where the country's minister of health also spoke.

It was exciting to see the critical mass of digital health forming and personally rewarding to feel I had contributed to it in small ways. Yet, as fascinating as the story of digital health is, in late 2016, while preparing for another keynote presentation, I had my second epiphany.

What follows is a treatise—or manifesto, if you will—on digital health. It serves as the foundation for my belief that the global impact of digital health is creating a new era of human progress. My hope is that readers from all backgrounds, representing all relevant stakeholder groups—consumers, business, technologists, scientists, policymakers, regulators, nongovernmental organizations (NGOs), and other institutions—will gain an understanding of the significance of what's happening, learn key actionable insights and, in the process, catalyze digital health, also known as the Fourth Wave.

Definition

To tell the story of digital health, it helps to begin with a definition. Simply put, digital health is the convergence of the Digital and Genomic Revolutions with health, healthcare, living, and society. This is necessarily a very broad definition, because digital technologies and, increasingly, genomic advancements, are touching, measuring, and impacting every aspect of our lives. As we are seeing and experiencing, digital health is empowering us to better track, manage, and improve our own and our families' health, live better, more productive lives, and improve society. It's also helping to reduce inefficiencies in healthcare delivery, improve access, reduce costs, increase quality, and make medicine more personalized and precise.

There are many examples of digital health we are all familiar with and use ourselves, including: tracking your workouts and nutrition with a smartphone app; using a heart rate monitor on your smartwatch or other fitness wearable; searching for fitness, health, medical information on the web (e.g. WebMD); using digital glucometers and continuous glucose monitors to help manage diabetes; participating in interactive (virtual or in-person) fitness classes that use your heart rate to optimize the workout for your body (e.g. Peloton and Orange Theory Fitness); speaking on your smartphone with your doctor, nurse, or other healthcare professional (including scheduling an appointment or consulting your doctor); accessing your healthcare records via the Internet; and even newborn genetic testing for identifying and treating diseases. The list goes on, and anyone can add to it very simply by using two simple criteria:

1. Is digital technology or genomics involved?
2. Is there an impact on human health, healthcare, living, or society?

Genomics

Up until the time that I expanded and promulgated a new definition of digital health, genomics was not considered part of the equation, but purely an area of biology and the life sciences. This is an oversight for a couple of reasons.

First, DNA is digital. Sometimes referred to as the blueprint or code of life, DNA contains all the necessary instructions for making a living organism, helping it survive, and reproducing it. Every single one of the living cells in your body contains this essential DNA code, which is comprised of 23 pairs of chromosomes. Half of these are inherited from your mother (in the egg), and half from your father (in the sperm). A genome is the total of our—or any organism's—DNA. We have an estimated 19,000 to 20,000 protein-coding genes in our chromosomes.

The word 'code' is not my choosing, but one used by scientists. Much like software code performs a function in a digital computer, DNA code performs the protein-coding function in our cells. However, unlike computer code—which is a binary code comprised of 1s and 0s—our DNA is comprised of a four-base code of chemicals, the nucleic acids adenine (A), cytosine (C), guanine (G), and thymine (T), aka ACGs and Ts.

In 1953, Francis Crick and James Watson identified the double-helix structure of the DNA molecule. Four years later, during a lecture on protein synthesis, Crick was the first to describe how the information in a gene is made up of this chemical code of four bases and that their sequence corresponds to the order of the amino acids in a resulting protein made in human cells. He called this the 'sequence hypothesis', likely leading to the modern terms we are familiar with: DNA sequencing and genome sequencing.

J. Craig Venter—who was one of the first to sequence the human genome, which he published in 2001—points out that the digital code and the genetic code have a lot in common: "We completely synthesized the genetic code of a cell starting with a digital code in the computer—it's the ultimate interface between computers and biology. The digital code and the genetic code have a lot in common; something Schrodinger pointed out in 1943, saying it could be something as simple as the Morse code. Digital code, as you know, is a binary code, and ones and zeroes, and your genetic code is literally four-base code with ACGs and Ts. We can now readily convert in between the two, and we can define life at its most basic level. Things that were a mystery fifty, sixty, seventy years ago, we now understand completely."

In a nutshell—or rather a human or any other living cell—the order of these chemical bases and how they pair up is what determine DNA's instructions, or genetic code. Our entire genome contains about 3 billion bases with, again around 20,000 or fewer of these being protein-coding genes. This equates to slightly more than 1 percent of our DNA coding for the proteins that determine much of the critical roles in our bodies, determining the structure, function, and regulation of our organs and tissues.

The second reason I include genomics in the definition of digital health is that the Digital Revolution—starting with digital electronics in the late 1950s—is both enabling and accelerating genomics well beyond what it otherwise would be as a field of science. Through the application of modern computing, next-generation sequencing (NGS) technologies, and robotics, the speed of genotyping (determining which genetic variants you possess) and genome sequencing (identifying the order of those four base pairs) has increased significantly over the past 16 years. In 2007, it may have taken 10 months to sequence a genome. Today it can take as little as just one hour.

And as the chart below illustrates, sequencing costs have even outpaced Moore's Law for computer processing speed. We are now at the point where DNA sequencing machines—like those produced by San Diego, CA-based Illumina—are delivering whole genome sequencing for just $1,000 per genome, and will soon do so for just $100.

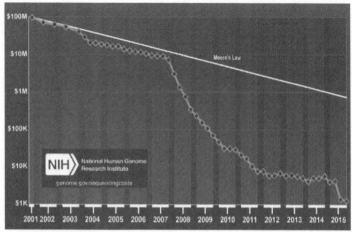

Figure 1: Cost to Sequence a Genome vs. Moore's Law of Computing Speed (Source: NHGRI)

As is typical when processes and systems become increasingly more computerized—in this case around an inherently digital input: DNA—the physical size of devices gets smaller. Genomics is experiencing this evolution, providing new opportunities for testing and sequencing to be performed in hospitals and doctor's offices, remote areas, desktop labs, even in the home, on the go (mobile devices) and, with real-time sequencing, as an element of the Internet of Things (IoT).

One example of this paradigm shift comes from DNA Electronics, which was founded in 2003 by Chris Toumazou, PhD, a professor at Imperial College London. The company's novel microchip technology can detect DNA nucleotides (ACGs and Ts) as electrical signals. Unlike current testing methods—for example those used to diagnose bloodstream infections leading to sepsis—

their LiDia genomic analysis system does not require a blood culture. As a result, diagnosis can take approximately 3 hours versus 1 to 6 days. According to DNA Electronics, sepsis is the leading cause of death from infection and cases have increased nearly 13% over the past decade, claiming more lives than bowel and breast cancer combined.

Another example is the MinION, a DNA analyzer and sequencer that fits in the palm of your hand. Made by Oxford Nanopore, the MinION can perform genetic testing as well as whole genome sequencing. The technology works by passing a DNA strand through a nano-scale hole (aka nanopore) that has an ionic current flowing through it. DNA nucleotides (ACGs and Ts) measurably change this current as they pass through the pore, enabling identification of molecules. Utilizing the MinION device, scientists recently turned a bus into a mobile genomics laboratory, driving it around the northeastern region of Brazil with the mission of finding mosquitoes infected with the Zika virus. By sequencing the Zika genome contained in the blood of collected mosquitoes, the scientists were able to study the evolution of the viral genome, thereby revealing vital clues about the origin of the epidemic. The pilot project also demonstrated the ability of the MinION to be used in the field, thereby eliminating the time-consuming process of sending samples back to a central lab for testing.

Lastly, you may wonder why I call it a Genomic Revolution versus a Genomics Revolution or a Genetics Revolution. First, while they are closely related, the fields of genomics and genetics are distinctly different.

According to the National Human Genome Research Institute (NHGRI), "Genetics is a term that refers to the study of genes and their roles in inheritance—in other words, the way that certain traits or conditions are passed down from one generation to another. Genetics involves scientific studies of genes and their effects. Genes (units of heredity) carry the instructions for making proteins, which direct the activities of cells and functions of the body. Examples of genetic or inherited disorders include cystic fibrosis."

Gregor Mendel is recognized as the founder of the science of genetics. As a result of his experiments with pea plants, Mendel established many of the rules of genetic heredity—now known as the laws of Mendelian inheritance—which he published in 1866. Mendel coined the terms 'recessive' and 'dominant' in regard to predictable genetic traits that were inherited by subsequent generations of pea plants. He described these inherited traits as being due to invisible factors, or what we now call genes.

The NHGRI also states that "Genomics—a more recent term—describes the study of all of a person's genes (the genome), including interactions of those genes with each other and with the person's environment. Genomics includes the scientific study of complex diseases such as heart disease, asthma, diabetes, and cancer because these diseases are typically caused more by a combination of genetic and environmental factors than by individual genes. Genomics is offering new possibilities for therapies and treatments for some complex diseases, as well as new diagnostic methods."

The wide-ranging perspective of genomics is essential to what we're seeing today in new and revolutionary scientific developments and applications. Genetics, with its narrower field of view, simply does not capture this panorama.

I use the term Genomic versus Genomics as a result of communications with entrepreneur Richard Resnick, whose 2016 TED Talk, 'Welcome to the Genomic Revolution' was an important influence on me. While formulating my definition for digital health, I reached out to Resnick and asked him why he chose to use the term 'genomic' versus 'genomics'. In an email to me, Resnick stated that "A 'Genomic Revolution' strikes me as more fundamental and powerful than a 'Genomics Revolution', because the latter seems to stress the technology behind the revolution, and the former is vamping more on the implicit societal change."

Resnick adds that when it comes to genetics vs. genomics, he feels that "The genetic revolution happened when we first started planting crops rather than gathering them, and when we first started cultivating wolves into dogs. And the Genomic Revolution implies an understanding of the genetic tOME—a totality of some sort—and is therefore analogous to the digital age. The idea behind the 'OME' is that of a totality of understanding, e.g., the biome as a totality of all living things, or a tome, which represents a very large volume of knowledge of some sort. So, we go from genetic—genesis, the beginning, etc., as being studied from the outside—to genome, the entirety of knowledge of genetics."

Looking at it another way, genomic (in reference to genomics) is similar to a panoramic view, in which we survey all aspects of a subject in a continuously passing or changing scene, or an unfolding of events. This is apropos the Genomic Revolution.

Cambrian Explosion

Digital health is currently experiencing its own version of the Cambrian explosion. Also known as the Cambrian period on Earth, the Cambrian explosion occurred around 540 million years ago during the Paleozoic Era. This was a relatively brief period of time—geologically speaking—of 50 million years (out of the Earth's 4.5 billion years), during which most of the major animal phyla appeared on the planet. Prior to this period, most organisms were simple, and made up only of individual cells that sometimes organized into colonies. During the Cambrian explosion—and over the course of the next 70-80 million—the rate of diversification of life on Earth accelerated by an order of magnitude, and the diversity of life began to resemble what we see today.

A similar situation is occurring in digital health, with the Digital Revolution now kicking into high gear and bringing into being a multitude of increasingly more sophisticated digital health innovations. Building upon the 'simple organisms' of the Digital Revolution—including microchips and computers, wireless networks, and the Internet—we're now seeing more complex digital organisms layered on top, including: more powerful and smaller computers, faster wireless networks, broadband, social networks. These have manifested into the major digital health phyla, including: smartphones and other mobile devices, wearable technology, sensors, robots, augmented reality (AR), virtual reality (VR), artificial intelligence (AI), and genomics.

Devices and Sensors

Wearable technology—like the Apple Watch and Fitbit—provides a variety of opportunities in digital health. This was highlighted by a survey of fitness industry professionals conducted by the American College of Sports Medicine (ACSM). These professionals indicated that the number one trend in their field for 2017 was wearable tech. Included by ACSM in this category are: activity trackers, smart watches, heart rate monitors, and GPS tracking devices. Also of relevance to digital health—and included in the top 20—were: Exercise as Medicine (an ACSM initiative focused on making exercise an integral part of healthcare), exercise and weight loss, fitness programs for older adults, worksite health promotion, smartphone exercise apps, and outcome measurements.

As the Mayo Clinic points out, wearable activity trackers and pedometers provide immediate feedback about your activity level and can serve as a strong motivator to keep you moving, while tracking your progress over time. Even simple nudges—like the Apple Watch's hourly alert to stand up—can provide a subtle but powerful tool for promoting physical activity, thereby reducing disease risk. Recently, many electronic health record (EHR) systems have been modified to allow for importing this type of consumer-generated health information. This enables doctors to monitor a patient's physical activity in a new, more precise way, thereby helping to improve the healthcare advice and services they provide.

Wearable devices and apps for health-tracking, sports, and fitness are in abundance these days. A recent review of several by Bloomberg reporter Aki Ito featured her take on 17 such products. While a personal fitness trainer in the video dismisses many of these as "tricks and tropes", Aki describes how one—the MOOV virtual fitness coach—appeared to have been effective in helping her achieve her goals, saying: "I lost almost seven pounds over the past three months, most of it in body fat, according to my Wi-Fi connected Body+ scale. I tried tracking my progress on a muscle-and-fat scanner called Skulpt, but its results were less conclusive, partly because the handheld scanning process was so time-consuming that I did it only sporadically. I feel stronger and lighter on my feet, and my clothes fit better. I ran a 1.5-mile sprint at the beginning and end of my project to test my cardiovascular strength, and I'm now more than a minute faster. I won't ever know if all that was because of the personal trainer or the wearables. As with most things in life, I'm sure it was a little bit of both."

As Aki notes, her attempt at measuring her body muscle and fat were unsuccessful. However, a consumer product called the Naked 3D Fitness Tracker offers a much more user-friendly method for accomplishing this. Comprised of a long mirror with embedded depth sensors—plus a Bluetooth-connected scale—the system captures a 3D model or your body, enabling you to visualize your body's changes over time using a companion app. The app also provides body weight, body measurements, and volumetric body fat percentage, in what is essentially a virtual hydrostatic (dunk tank) test. There's even a body 'heat map', which indicates the specific locations where you are growing muscle or gaining fat.

Modern wearable devices are increasingly filled with all types of sensors, including: accelerometer, heart rate sensor, GPS, gyroscope, compass, microphone, light, barometer, altimeter, camera, and temperature. While accelerometers, heart rate, and temperature (thermometer) sensors have obvious applications for health, there are many ingenious uses for other sensors, not to mention the capacity to derive valuable health-related information by correlating data from multiple sensors and other data sources. One example by Senosis Health—a startup company recently acquired by Verily (an Alphabet subsidiary, also Google's parent company), utilizes smartphone sensors to measure blood hemoglobin and identify jaundice in newborns (using the camera), measure lung function (using the microphone), and bone strength (using accelerometers).

And new nanotube sensors under development offer the potential for being introduced into the blood or implanted in the body, where they could track insulin levels, the blood-clotting protein fibrinogen, or even nitric oxide, a signaling molecule associated with many cancer cells. The system works as a result of the nanotubes fluorescing when they bind to molecules of interest. This can then be detected in a blood sample or by placing a light-emitting wireless patch on the skin above the embedded nanotube sensor. This data can, in turn, be transmitted to a smartphone and healthcare provider for real-time monitoring and early intervention to better manage, diagnose, or prevent disease.

Apps and Social Media

We all have our favorite apps on our smartphones and computers: be they email, maps and navigational aids, nutrition and fitness tracking, restaurant information, banking and of course, social networking apps like Facebook, Instagram, Snapchat, and Twitter. While our experiences with these platforms are mostly positive— bringing us closer to friends and family, making new connections, joining like-minded communities, navigating to a destination, learning new things—there can be downsides.

Research shows that we touch, swipe, or tap our phones more than 2,600 times a day. And it's no wonder this so-called 'smartphone addiction' occurs, as app features—such as the 'like' button on Facebook, Instagram, and Twitter—trigger a jolt of dopamine that's sent to the brain's reward and pleasure centers. Other features—which are purposely designed to keep us engaged on the app platforms—include notifications, video autoplay, and pull-to-refresh features. This ongoing digital assault limits our ability to focus and can possibly lower IQ. A recent study suggests that even the mere presence of a smartphone damages our cognitive capacity. According to Justin Rosenstein, a Facebook engineer who co-created the 'like' button, "Everyone is distracted all of the time."

A recent study on the impact of social networking apps on young people's mental health conducted by the Royal Society for Public Health revealed some troubling issues. Teens and young adults were surveyed and asked questions revealing issues around anxiety, depression, self-identity, and body image. While YouTube was found to have a net positive impact, apps like Instagram, Snapchat, Facebook and Twitter all demonstrated negative affects overall on young people's mental health. Instagram—the image-sharing app with over 700 million users—ranked worst in terms of negative impact, particularly among young women. According to study author Matt Keracher, the app leads young women to "compare themselves against unrealistic, largely curated, filtered, and Photoshopped versions of reality." One anonymous female respondent stated that "Instagram easily makes girls and women feel as if their bodies aren't good enough, as people add filters and edit their pictures in order for them to look 'perfect'."

Psychologists are also seeing that digital technology is causing loneliness in adolescents and teenagers. One study found that approximately 6% of adolescents and teens engage in 'digital self-harm', which is the practice of posting or sharing demeaning information about oneself anonymously online. Justin Patchin, lead author of the study, said that he was surprised that the numbers were as high as they were. And Danah Boyd, PhD, a digital self-harm researcher and author of 'It's Complicated: The Social Lives of Networked Teens', states "I don't think it dawned on anyone that teens would leverage anonymity in this way. It tends to startle anyone I tell about it." While digital self-harm can validate a young person's insecurities, it can also serve as way to purge bad self-impressions by safely obtaining attention from friends about the negative feelings they have inside.

In light of these downsides of social media and smartphone use, particularly for teens, it was fascinating to see that Facebook recently acquired a 'positively-focused' anonymous teen compliment app named tbh. In just over two months, the app had 5 million downloads and 2.5 million daily users, who use it to anonymously answer 'kind-hearted' multiple-choice questions about their friends. The results are then sent to their friends as compliments. According to tbh co-creator Nikita Bier, "If we're improving the mental health of millions of teens, that's a success to us."

When it comes to online dating apps, recent research has found that they are even changing the nature of society in a couple of key ways. Dating websites—like Match.com, Tinder, and OKCupid—are changing the way couples meet, which is influencing the levels of interracial marriage and the stability of marriage itself. Incredibly, more than 33% of marriages are now the result of couples who met online. Evidence shows that these marriages are stronger and have lower rates of marital breakup than marriages beginning from traditional ways of meeting. And with racial diversity being a key metric of social distance, interracial marriage can provide a major benefit to society. Interestingly, "Swipe Right," a new comedy series about dating using the Tinder app (and based on a true story by lead actress Carly Craig) is set to air in 2018 on online video platform YouTube Red.

In 2015, IMS Health (now IQVIA) identified more than 165,000 health and fitness apps in the mobile app stores, a number equivalent to about 8.6% of all apps at the time. In looking at a sample of 26,000 of these apps, the report identified that 36 accounted for 50% of downloads, 10% connected to a device or sensor, and 34% connected to social networks. Also, 85% focused on wellness and disease management, with the remaining 15% focused on providing health information.

In January of 2017, I looked at the top apps in the 'Health & Fitness' section of the Apple iTunes app store. Eight of the top nine fall within the 'wellness and disease management' category: MyFitnessPal, Fitbit, Lose It! Calorie Counter, Map My Run by Under Armour, Weight Watchers, Nike+ Run Club, Period Tracker Lite, and Runkeeper. The ninth, WebMD, falls within the 'health information' category. I took a second look at the top apps in November 2017 and the standings had not changed. The tenth most popular app was Headspace, a meditation and mindfulness app that has been downloaded more than 11 million times as of January 2017, plus has nearly half a million paid subscribers. This is significant for a couple of reasons: It's a large number of people and, as indicated four paragraphs below, a recent study of mindfulness apps has shown that they can help people with mild-to-moderate levels of depression.

In November 2017, IQVIA updated their analysis of health apps and expanded their focus to also include consumer wearable tech devices. The company identified 318,000 health-related mobile applications available to consumers in the app stores—nearly double the number in 2015. Similar to 2015, when just 36 apps accounted for 50% of downloads, in 2017 just 41 apps (with over 10 million downloads each) accounted for nearly half of all downloads.

According to the report: "This rapid app expansion, coupled with more than 340 consumer wearable devices on the market worldwide, provide evidence of digital health's accelerating innovation. At this time, there is at least one high-quality app for each step of the patient journey. While the majority of mobile health apps available are general wellness apps, the number of health condition management apps—those often associated with patient care—are increasing at a faster rate, and now represent 40 percent of all health-related apps."

IQVIA further indicates that: "The overall body of clinical evidence on app efficacy has grown substantially and now includes 571 published studies, enabling the identification of a list of top apps with increasingly robust clinical evidence." Moreover, the report suggests that the use of digital health apps and wearables in just five patient populations where they have proven reductions in acute care utilization—diabetes prevention, diabetes, asthma, cardiac rehabilitation, and pulmonary rehabilitation—could save the U.S. healthcare system an estimated $7 billion per year, or about 1.4% of total costs in these patient populations, adding that if these savings are extrapolated across all disease areas, an annual cost savings of $46 billion could be achieved.

Apps in the wellness category can also provide surprising benefits for mental health. Researchers in Australia found that smartphone apps focused on mindfulness, cognitive behavioral therapy, and mood altering programs can help with mild-to-moderate levels of depression. Interestingly, self-contained apps outperformed combination therapies, i.e. apps integrating computer and human clinician feedback. The authors suggest that the comprehensiveness of stand-alone apps may explain their superior results. Study coauthor John Torous, MD, who is co-director of the digital psychiatry program at Beth Israel Deaconess Medical Center, stated that "Patients and doctors are faced with a vast array of mental health apps these days, and knowing which ones are actually helpful is imperative. This research provides much needed information on the effectiveness of apps for depression, and offers important clues into the types of apps which can help patients manage their condition."

Social media is also having a unique impact on politics and the media. In a recent interview, Glenn Greenwald, an editor and journalist with The Intercept, stated that there is a "Very severe groupthink that social media is fostering in ways that we don't yet fully understand. Most journalists these days aren't in Congressional Committees or at zoning board meetings, or using shoe-leather reporting—they're sitting on Twitter talking to one another and this produces this extreme groupthink where these orthodoxies arise and deviating from them or questioning them or challenging—believe me—results in all kinds of recrimination and scorn. And embracing them produces this sort of in-group mentality where you are rewarded, and I think a lot of it is about that kind of behavior."

Greenwald adds that, "Because what you see is over and over they (journalists) publish really inflammatory stories that turn out to be totally false and what happens in those cases? Nothing. They get enormous benefits when they publish recklessly. They get applause on social media from their peers, they get zillions of re-tweets, huge amounts of traffic, they end up on TV. They get applauded across the spectrum because people are so giddy and eager to hear more about this Russia and Trump story."

More recently, in reference to the political controversy involving Donna Brazile and the Democratic National Committee, plus documents and emails published by WikiLeaks during the 2016 presidential campaign, Greenwald pointed out four major factually false claims that went viral as a result of journalists on Twitter endorsing and spreading them. Reemphasizing his previous comments about the power of social media: "Claims from journalists that people want to believe are shared like wildfire, while less popular, subsequent corrections or nuanced debunking are easily ignored. Whatever one's views are on the actual impact of Twitter Russian bots, surely the propensity of journalistic falsehoods to spread far and wide is at least as significant."

The obsessive focus on viewer traffic (a key metric for increasing advertising revenue) was on glaring display in the 2016 U.S. Presidential election. Speaking candidly about Donald Trump's candidacy, Leslie Moonves, CEO at CBS—a mass media corporation focused on commercial broadcasting, publishing, and television production—stated: "It may not be good for America, but it's damn good for CBS. Man, who would have expected the ride we're all having right now? The money's rolling in and this is fun. I've never seen anything like this, and this (is) going to be a very good year for us. Sorry. It's a terrible thing to say. But, bring it on, Donald. Keep going."

CBS was not alone in this frenzy, as it was reported that Donald Trump benefited from $5.6 billion in free 'earned' media coverage during the election season. This amount was greater than that received by all the other candidates combined: Hillary Clinton, Bernie Sanders, Ted Cruz, Paul Ryan, and Marco Rubio. Rather than paying for advertising, the Trump campaign received free mentions on major TV news networks, online media, and social media. For example, on Twitter, where Trump received 150% more coverage than Clinton, his 'taco bowl tweet' generated nearly $200 million in free attention alone.

On the flipside, according to The Guardian's Ben Tarnoff, social media is helping emerging movements unite against the elites. Tarnoff states that social media isn't just a tool for mobilizing people—exemplified by the networked uprisings of 2011 (the year of the Arab spring, Occupy Wall Street, and the Spanish anti-austerity Indignados movements)—it's also a tool for politicizing them. Tarnoff adds that: "The mainstream media tends to be hostile to the left: proximity to power often leads journalists to internalize the perspectives of society's most powerful people. The result is a public sphere that sets narrow parameters for permissible political discourse, and ignores or vilifies those who step outside of them. That's why social media is indispensable: it provides a space for incubating new kinds of political thinking, and new forms of political identity, that would be inadmissible in more established channels."

While the examples I've highlighted may skew towards the downsides of apps, social media, and the Internet, these digital tools and platforms will continue to be both inescapable and essential components of living in modern society. As such, it's critical that we have balanced, objective, and realistic perspectives, and not focus only on the positive benefits they provide.

Internet access—which has become comparable to public utilities like running water and electricity—is considered to be such a vital aspect of society that more than 70 countries now consider it a basic human right for their citizens. In light of this, it's not too surprising that, in 2016, the United Nations Human Rights Council passed a non-binding resolution that condemns any countries that take away or disrupt Internet access for their citizens.

As with previous technology-driven sociocultural evolutions, along with positive advances also come downsides, including: economic dislocation; consolidation of wealth and power; and loss of independence, privacy, and individuality. While society moves forward, it can leave some people and groups behind, even as the benefits accrue to society as a whole. Therefore, it's important that we have monitoring, checks and balances, and focus on democratization and the equitable distribution of gains, while concurrently striving to reduce the negative impacts.

Key Factors

While digital health has been around for decades—for example, electronic health records and the wearable Holter Monitor for heart monitoring were developed in the 1960s—there are a variety of key factors accelerating digital health at this time. These include the economics of healthcare costs and access to healthcare, investing and innovation acceleration, regulation, and market opportunities. All are intrinsically linked and mutually-amplifying of each other.

Economics and Access

The cost of healthcare and resulting financial burdens placed on the federal government, consumers (households), private businesses, and state & local governments continues to rise faster than the rate of inflation. In 2015, total spending on healthcare in the United States amounted to $3.2 trillion. This represented an increase of 5.8% from 2014 and an incredible 17.8% of the nation's gross domestic product (GDP). Looked at another way, this is equivalent to about $10,000 per person living in the United States.

Health Spending by Stakeholder Group (2015)

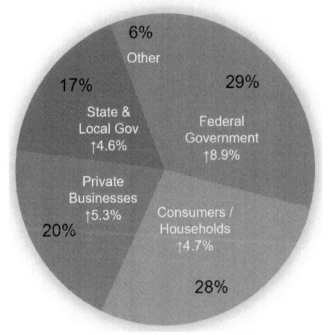

Figure 2: Health Spending by Stakeholder Group (Source: CMS & Paul Sonnier)

Since 1980, spending on healthcare as a percentage of gross domestic product (GDP), has increased in most major economies, not just the United States. However, spending has grown the fastest and is the largest in the U.S., with cost burden falling on the shoulders of consumers and employers increasing nearly 60% since 2006. Because of this critical situation, one of the main objectives of the Affordable Care Act (ACA)— aka Obamacare—was to lower the costs of healthcare generally. The ACA also sought to increase the number of Americans with health insurance. According to the Kaiser Family Foundation, the number of uninsured nonelderly Americans decreased from 44 million in 2013 (the year before the major ACA coverage provisions went into effect) to 28 million as of the end of 2016.

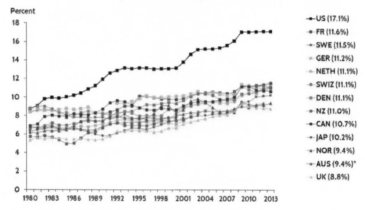

Figure 3: Health Care Spending as a Percentage of GDP (Source: OECD & Commonwealth Fund)

In 2015, the World Health Organization (WHO) and the World Bank estimated that 400 million people worldwide lacked access to at least one of seven essential health services, ranging from pregnancy care to clean water. Exacerbating the problem, the current global healthcare workforce shortage is projected to worsen, reaching 12.9 million workers by 2035. In the U.S., the Association of American Medical Colleges (AAMC) predicts a shortage of nearly 100,000 physicians by 2025. These healthcare provider shortages represent serious implications for the health of billions of people around the world.

The WHO also indicates that almost 2% of people have experienced catastrophic healthcare spending, which is defined as being equivalent to costs totaling more than 25% of household expenditures. And 17% of households tipped or fell even further below the extreme poverty line (income of $2 per day) because of healthcare costs. The report went on to add that universal health coverage—while controversial—is achievable, and would undoubtedly address this problem.

A major factor in the high cost of healthcare in the United States is the cost of drugs. Many life-saving drugs are half the cost in Canada and Europe versus the U.S., according to economist Dean Baker, co-director of the Center for Economic and Policy Research (CEPR). Baker adds that drug patents are part of the problem, stating that: "There are no government granted patent monopolies in a free market. As a result of these government granted monopolies, we will pay more than $440 billion for prescription drugs this year. These drugs would likely cost less than $80 billion in a free market. The difference of more than $360 billion a year is a bit less than 2% of GDP." Baker adds that "The same story applies to medical equipment. MRIs are cheap without patent protection. It is possible to argue for the merits of government granted monopolies (I argue against them in chapter 5 of (his book) "Rigged: How Globalization and the Rules of the Modern Economy Were Structured to Make the Rich Richer"), but it is not possible to deny that these monopolies are a government policy, not the free market."

Reinforcing Baker's points about high drug prices and their contribution to healthcare costs, when the FDA approved PCSK9 inhibitors, a new class of drugs intended to treat high cholesterol, Bernard J. Tyson, Chairman and CEO of the Kaiser Foundation Health Plan and Hospitals, highlighted that this would be the most expensive class of drugs ever, and "threatens to undermine the health care system upon which the drug industry relies." In a 2015 Forbes op-ed 'Why Pharma Must Change Its Model', Tyson adds that: "The average American family pays the healthcare industry about $25,000 every year. In return, they expect us to deliver all of their care—including medical advances. It's a more than reasonable expectation. There is no question that we should be able to solve our healthcare problems for well within the 18% of GDP that goes towards it. Every part of the industry has been shaken up by this new era of doing better for less. Countless industries outside of health care have already gone before us, understanding that technology and productivity gains must be passed along to the consumer for businesses and our nation to remain competitive. The pharmaceutical industry remains our lone holdout, and we cannot succeed without it. If the cost of new drugs continues to rise at this rate, any progress we make in other parts of the health ecosystem will be irrelevant."

Another contributing factor to high healthcare costs is that, unlike most developed countries, the U.S. does not have a single-payer, universal healthcare system. As Robert H. Frank, professor of economics at

Cornell University explains his New York Times op-ed, 'Why Single-Payer Health Care Saves Money', insurance reform—in the form of a single-payer system—would substantially lower the total cost of healthcare delivery. Professor Frank writes that "Sometimes described as Medicare for all, single-payer is a system in which a public agency handles health care financing while the delivery of care remains largely in private hands. As experience in many countries has demonstrated, the total cost of providing health coverage under the single-payer approach is actually substantially lower than under the current system in the United States."

During a speech in November 2017, former United Nations secretary general Ban Ki-moon called on Americans to pass universal health coverage. He stated that powerful interests are prioritizing profit over care and preventing the adoption of a publicly financed health system similar to those used in other wealthy countries. "In the U.S.," Ki-moon states, "all too often only rich people get access to expensive life-saving treatments. This is unjust and threatens everybody's health when working- and middle-class people with communicable diseases cannot afford treatment for their infections. Even routine preventive care is often prohibitively expensive. As America is demonstrating, you simply cannot reach universal health coverage if your health system is dominated by private financing and ultimately functions to prioritize profit over care."

And doctor salaries, as well, are another significant contributor to the high cost of healthcare in the United States. Dean Baker points out that, on average, U.S. doctors are paid twice as much as physicians in other wealthy countries, resulting in $100 billion per year more in healthcare costs. He says this is due in large part to a form of trade protectionism enjoyed by our doctors, which protects them from both foreign and domestic competition. Foreign doctors are currently prohibited from practicing in the U.S. unless they complete a U.S. residency program. And foreign dentists—except for those trained in Canadian schools—are prohibited from practicing in the U.S. unless they graduate from a U.S. dental school. Moreover, the number of residency slots available for training new doctors has been frozen since 1997, when the U.S. Congress lowered the number at the request of the American Medical Association (AMA) and other organizations that represent doctors.

Baker suggests some ways to address this cost premium, including allowing foreign medical schools to be certified to train doctors to practice here, allowing foreign-trained doctors to practice under the supervision of U.S. doctors (as a few states are already testing), and increasing the number of medical residency slots while allotting a greater percentage to training general practitioners versus higher-paid specialists (two-thirds of U.S. doctors are specialists, as compared to one-third in most other wealthy countries). He adds that permitting nurse practitioners to perform more procedures and prescribing medicine without a doctor's supervision (as many states are already doing) would also help drive down costs.

A relevant example of the potential for digital health to reduce these costs was highlighted in a recent NPR piece, which pointed out that radiologists—who make $400,000 per year, on average—see their jobs at risk due to 'machines'. According to radiology fellow Phelps Kelley, MD, "The biggest concern is that we could be replaced by machines. Radiology has become commoditized over the years. People don't want interaction with a radiologist, they just want a piece of paper that says what the CT (computed tomography) shows." Bob Wachter, MD—author of 'The Digital Doctor: Hope, Hype, and Harm at the Dawn of Medicine's Computer Age'—echoes this point, stating that: "Radiology, at its core, is now a human being, based on learning and his or her own experience, looking at a collection of digital dots and a digital pattern and saying 'That pattern looks like cancer or looks like tuberculosis or looks like pneumonia. Computers are awfully good at seeing patterns."

So where does all of this leave us? Simply put— though not simply accomplished—radically transforming U.S. healthcare to deliver the best quality of care and in the most cost-efficient manner requires a multifaceted approach. This includes continued adoption of digital health, a single-payer, universal health coverage system (for example, the Medicare for All plan proposed by Senator Bernie Sanders (I-VT)), drug-price negotiation, pharmaceutical and medical device industry patent reform, publicly financed pharmaceutical research and clinical trials, and addressing the systemic issues causing high doctor salaries.

Investing and Innovation Acceleration

Investment in digital health innovation—particularly solutions being developed and commercialized by startup companies—has been booming for several years. In 2016, over 900 global entities invested in more than 500 deals, with a combined value of more than $8 billion. This represents a 730% increase since 2010. According to Startup Health—an innovation accelerator with a portfolio of more than 180 digital health companies—as of September of 2017, digital health funding year to date (YTD) surpassed $9 billion, exceeding the total for all of 2016. The organization predicts that funding in 2017 will reach or exceed a record $10 billion.

Notably, in the years 2014 and 2016, digital health venture capital (VC) investing overtook venture capital investing in biotech. This is an indication of the value proposition of digital health and that, in some cases, private equity investors see startups in digital health as offering greater return on investment potential than startups in the biotech sector.

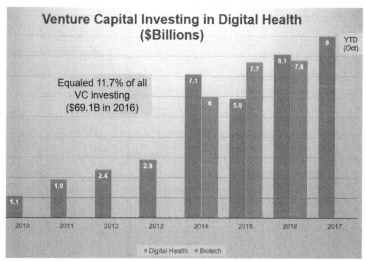

Figure 4: Venture Capital Investing in Digital Health (Source: StartUp Health and Paul Sonnier)

In 2015, StartUp Health estimated that there were approximately 8,000 startups focused on digital health located around the globe. On my website, I've compiled a searchable and filterable list of just over 700 entities (startups, established companies, and other organizations) that are developing and selling digital health solutions.

There are also a wide variety of innovation acceleration efforts underway around the world. By my count, there are over 30 standalone digital health organizations and institutes focused on digital health and more than 80 startup accelerators and incubators. And as of 2017, nearly 75% of large healthcare organizations have either built a digital health innovation center or have plans to do so soon.

Regulation

The U.S. Food and Drug Administration (FDA) is the main federal agency responsible for protecting the public health by assuring the safety, efficacy, and security of human and veterinary drugs, biological products, medical devices, the food supply, cosmetics, and products that emit radiation. Like many other organizations are now doing since I started promulgating a modernized definition of digital health, the FDA uses the term, and has even created a web page with a definition validating my own definition and benefits statement for digital health.

In a June 2017 post, FDA commissioner Scott Gottlieb, MD, described the agency's plans for a major initiative focused on fostering new innovation across its medical product centers, with a critical aspect being a Digital Health Innovation Plan. The plan, he said, would include a "novel, post-market approach to how we intend to regulate these digital medical devices." The intent, he added, is for developers to apply the FDA regulatory scheme on their own versus having to seek out the agency's "position on every individual technological change or iterative software development."

In August 2017 the FDA formally announced this Digital Health Innovation Action Plan and the launch of a Software Precertification (PreCert) Pilot Program, stating: "Digital health technology has become a new health care revolution that empowers consumers to make better-informed decisions about their health. At the FDA, we recognize this revolution and are reimagining our oversight of digital health technology to help provide patients with timely access to high-quality, safe, and effective digital health products. We've provided details and timelines for our digital health efforts in our Digital Health Innovation Action Plan, and one important piece of this plan is a new pilot program for software developers."

Bakul Patel, associate director for digital health at CDRH, highlighted the agency's stated digital health mission and regulatory transformation efforts, saying in a recent interview: "We've been trying to translate the current regulation paradigm for digital, but what we have today and what we're going to have tomorrow are not really translatable. We need to take the blinders off, start with a clean sheet of paper. The idea is to get safe products to market faster, by having people compete on excellence rather than compliance. We're headed toward a zero-code world, where AI writes it for you or you just say what you want and natural language processing takes care of the rest. The pace will be tremendously faster than what we're seeing today. The question is, how do we align our regulations to that radically different development timeline?"

Outside observers are also acknowledging the FDA's digital health efforts. As Bradley Merrill Thompson, an attorney with Epstein Becker & Green and head of the Clinical Decision Support Coalition, a digital health industry group, states: "Why the favorable regulatory environment for digital health? Quite honestly because many people at FDA see great public health benefits to these technologies. This is frankly the most excited we've ever seen the FDA. They truly want to foster safe innovation that leads to better clinical and patient reported outcomes."

As part of the Digital Health Innovation Action Plan, in September 2017, the FDA selected nine participants for a new Digital Health Precertification Pilot Program: Apple, Fitbit, Johnson & Johnson, Pear Therapeutics, Phosphorus, Roche, Samsung, Tidepool, and Verily. The list includes startups, large corporations, and nonprofit organizations that produce high- and low-risk medical device software products. According to an FDA announcement, the program is intended to inform a tailored approach toward digital health technology by looking at the software developer or digital health technology developer, rather than primarily at the product. The goal of this new approach is for the FDA to, after reviewing systems for software design, validation and maintenance, determine whether the company meets quality standards and if so, to precertify the company. With the information gleaned through the pilot program, the agency hopes to determine the key metrics and performance indicators for precertification and identify ways that precertified companies could potentially submit less information to the FDA than is currently required before marketing a new digital health tool as part of a formal program. The FDA is also considering, as part of the pilot program, whether and how precertified companies may not have to submit a product for premarket review in some cases.

In November 2017, the FDA's digital health precertification approach was expanded to cover direct-to-consumer (DTC) genomic tests for health risks. According to FDA commissioner Gottlieb: "At a time when people are more aware of and engaged in their health care than ever before, genetic risk testing can provide helpful information about an individual's predisposition for certain diseases and conditions. These tests can prompt consumers to be more engaged in pursuing the benefits of healthy lifestyle choices and more aware of their health risks. Consumers are increasingly embracing genetic health risk (GHR) testing to better understand their individual risk for developing diseases. This engagement prompts some people to make more informed lifestyle choices. Direct-to-consumer (DTC) access to GHR tests is made possible by advances in technology. With a small saliva sample, consumers can retrieve their genetic risk result directly from the test provider's website. As consumer interest in genetic risk information grows, opportunities are also expanding for the detection of additional genetic conditions and diseases that can help inform people of their medical risks."

As part of this new regulatory approach for DTC genomic testing, the FDA will exempt GHR tests from premarket review under certain conditions. Manufacturers must first submit to a one-time review to ensure that they meet the agency's requirements, after which they can introduce new GHR tests without further review. The agency also exempted genetic carrier screening tests from premarket review.

The FDA has recently approved several noteworthy new genetic tests and other types of digital health solutions:

- In April 2017, prior to the FDA's new DTC genetic health risk testing regulatory approach, the agency approved a total of ten GHR tests from 23andMe. In its announcement, the FDA stated that these tests work by isolating DNA from a saliva sample, which is then tested for more than 500,000 genetic variants. The presence or absence of some of these variants is associated with an increased risk for developing any one of the following 10 diseases or conditions:
  - Parkinson's disease: A nervous system disorder impacting movement
  - Late-onset Alzheimer's disease: A progressive brain disorder that destroys memory and thinking skills
  - Celiac disease: A disorder resulting in the inability to digest gluten
  - Alpha-1 antitrypsin deficiency: A disorder that raises the risk of lung and liver disease
  - Early-onset primary dystonia: A movement disorder involving involuntary muscle contractions and other uncontrolled movements
  - Factor XI deficiency: A blood clotting disorder
  - Gaucher disease type 1: An organ and tissue disorder

- o Glucose-6-Phosphate Dehydrogenase deficiency (G6PD): A red blood cell condition
- o Hereditary hemochromatosis: An iron overload disorder
- o Hereditary thrombophilia: A blood clot disorder
- A de novo (first of its kind) approval for a prescription digital therapeutic from Pear Therapeutics. The company's reSET system is used in the treatment of patients with substance use disorder (SUD) to help improve clinical outcomes when used in conjunction with standard outpatient treatment for SUDs related to stimulants, cannabis, cocaine, and alcohol. However, it is not intended to be used to treat opioid dependence.
- Abbott's FreeStyle Libre Flash wearable device and app system used for continuous glucose monitoring (CGM). Unlike competitor Dexcom's CGM system, the Abbott solution does not require calibration via fingerprick blood draws, which is a first for this type of digital health solution. According to the FDA's Donald St. Pierre: "This system allows people with diabetes to avoid the additional step of fingerstick calibration, which can sometimes be painful, but still provides necessary information for treating their diabetes—with a wave of the mobile reader."
- The first over-the-counter (OTC) carbon monoxide breath sensor system for use in

smoking cessation programs. Made by Carrot, Inc., the wireless device measures carbon monoxide in exhaled breath and, via a smartphone app, informs the user about how breath carbon monoxide levels are affected by smoking behavior. As with fitness wearables for tracking metrics like steps and sleep, the breath sensor enables a user to track the real-time effects of their smoking behavior to help them overcome their addiction.

- A virtual reality (VR) rehab device for stroke and brain injury patients made by MindMaze. The company's neurotechnology platform creates a virtual environment containing 3D avatars (linked to a patient's movements) and leads them through rehabilitation exercises.

- On November 13, 2017, the FDA approved Otsuka Pharmaceutical's Abilify MyCite, a pill with a sensor inside that digitally tracks when patients have ingested the medication. The pill is approved for the treatment of schizophrenia, acute treatment of manic and mixed episodes associated with bipolar I disorder, and for use as an add-on treatment for depression in adults. The system works by sending a message from the pill's sensor to a wearable patch, which then transmits information to a mobile app that enables patients to track ingestion of the medication. It also allows patients to share this information with their caregivers and physicians. The ingestible sensor used in the pill is made by Proteus Digital Health and was first permitted for marketing by the FDA in 2012.

Another United States federal regulatory agency actively involved in digital health is the Federal Trade Commission (FTC). The agency provides an interactive tool for developers of health apps that collect, create, or share consumer information. The tool is intended to help developers better understand when the FDA, FTC, and the Office of Civil Rights (OCR) laws apply to their products.

The FTC is also involved in enforcement when it comes to apps that cross the line by making unproven health or medical claims. In 2011, the agency fined the makers of two apps that claimed to cure acne via light emitted from a smartphone screen. And in 2014, the FTC brought a case against GeneLink, a direct-to-consumer (DTC) genetic testing company that claimed its DNA tests were able to identify a person's genetic weaknesses and cure them with dietary supplements and a genetically-personalized skin serum.

Markets

The market opportunities for digital health are diverse and spread across all major sectors of the economy, generally falling within the following categories and approximate sizes: health and fitness ($3.8 trillion); healthcare ($18.5 trillion); clinical trials and pharmaceuticals ($1.3 trillion); and other/related sectors ($18.6 trillion). The combined total is approximately $43 trillion. Also of significant relevance is agriculture, which is discussed in a later section.

These estimated market values are obtained from various sources. There are also overlaps. My main intent here is to provide a frame of reference on the aggregate size of relevant market opportunities for digital health and related solutions. The total addressable market (TAM) for digital health is of variable size within each market category.

The total of $43 trillion puts into perspective and validates the anticipated $10 billion that investors are expected to put towards funding of digital health startups and initiatives.

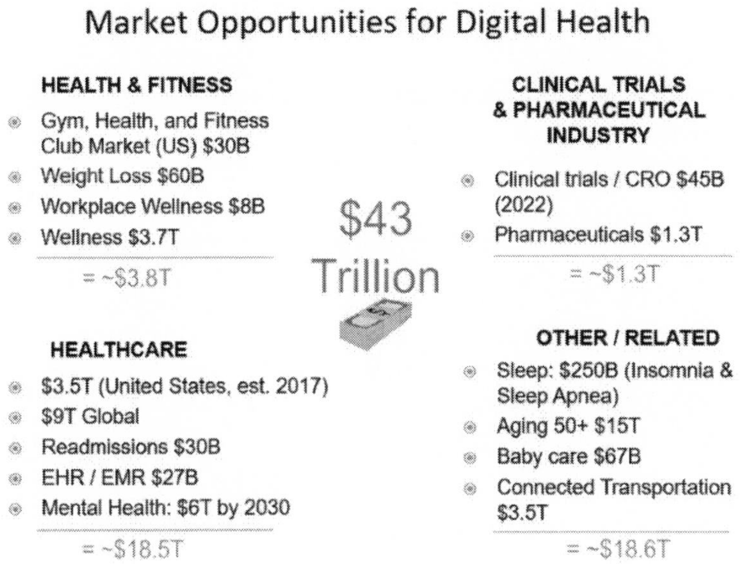

Market Opportunities for Digital Health

HEALTH & FITNESS

- Gym, Health, and Fitness Club Market (US) $30B
- Weight Loss $60B
- Workplace Wellness $8B
- Wellness $3.7T

= ~$3.8T

HEALTHCARE

- $3.5T (United States, est. 2017)
- $9T Global
- Readmissions $30B
- EHR / EMR $27B
- Mental Health: $6T by 2030

= ~$18.5T

$43 Trillion

CLINICAL TRIALS & PHARMACEUTICAL INDUSTRY

- Clinical trials / CRO $45B (2022)
- Pharmaceuticals $1.3T

= ~$1.3T

OTHER / RELATED

- Sleep: $250B (Insomnia & Sleep Apnea)
- Aging 50+ $15T
- Baby care $67B
- Connected Transportation $3.5T

= ~$18.6T

Figure 5: Market Opportunities for Digital Health (Source: Paul Sonnier)

Strategies

New technologies and derived innovations resulting from the Digital Revolution continue to disrupt traditional industries and ways of doing business. Clayton Christensen—author of the 1997 book 'The Innovator's Dilemma: When New Technologies Cause Great Firms to Fail'—points out that established companies can miss out on new waves of innovation (like digital health) unless their leaders and managers know when to abandon traditional business practices. Products and services, he says, take root initially in simple applications at the bottom of a market, then move up market, and eventually displace established competitors.

Two notable examples cited by Christensen are personal computers, which disrupted mainframe computers, and cellular phones, which disrupted fixed-line telephones. More recent examples include Uber disrupting the taxi industry; Amazon and Alibaba (ecommerce) disrupting traditional, brick-and-mortar retailers and booksellers; and Airbnb disrupting the hotel and accommodation industry. Moreover, Netflix displaced Blockbuster and Disney acquired Pixar Animation Studios to remain competitive in the animated movie business. At the time, the $7.4 billion acquisition was described by the Associated Press as putting "Steve Jobs in (a) powerful role as entertainment goes digital".

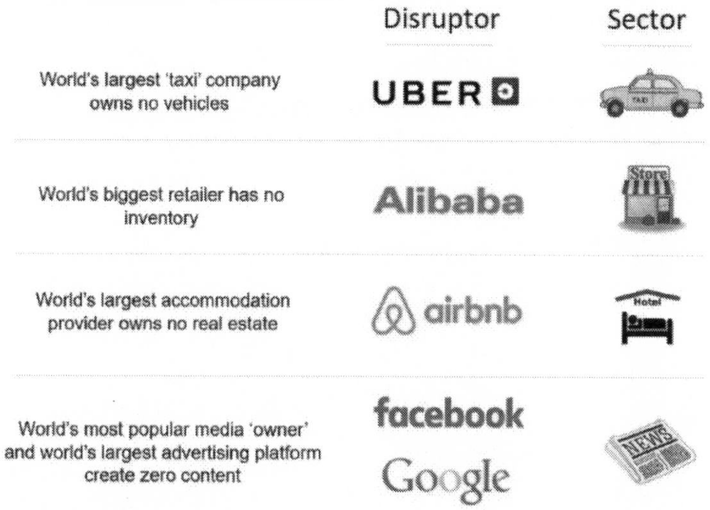

	Disruptor	Sector
World's largest 'taxi' company owns no vehicles	**UBER⊡**	
World's biggest retailer has no inventory	**Alibaba**	
World's largest accommodation provider owns no real estate	**airbnb**	
World's most popular media 'owner' and world's largest advertising platform create zero content	**facebook** Google	

Figure 6: Examples of Disruption (Source: Tom Goodwin & Paul Sonnier)

Disruption is not always a process consisting of new entrants—operating within the boundaries of an industry or sector—displacing incumbents. Sometimes disruption occurs exogenously, as the result of new or even existing entrants operating outside of an established sector. One of the best examples of this occurred in—or rather *to*—the newspaper industry. As the graph below illustrates, shortly after Google was founded it began generating significant amounts of advertising revenue. The search engine became an advertising platform, much like newspapers. But unlike newspapers, Google does not produce its own news content. Nonetheless, the company diverted the main source of revenue—advertising dollars—away from the newspaper industry by providing a digital customer interface comprised of high-intent users seeking out very specific products, services, and topics. Google offered a way for advertisers to target this demand. Print newspapers simply could not compete with Google's platform, and the industry's primary source of revenue was disrupted.

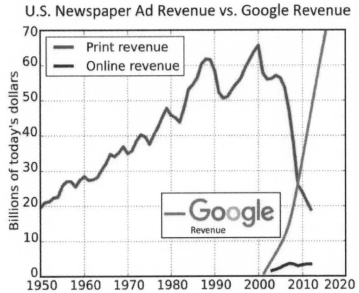

Figure 7: U.S. Newspaper Ad Revenue vs. Google Revenue (Source: Newspaper Association of America, Dave Farrance, & Paul Sonnier)

Steve Case—who cofounded America Online (AOL) in 1985—was one of the pioneers of the Internet. In his 2016 book, 'The Third Wave: An Entrepreneur's Vision of the Future', Case describes how AOL and other companies—including IBM, Apple, Cisco, Sun Microsystems, and Sprint—helped build the Internet and lay the foundation for consumers to connect to it. He describes this period (1985-1999) as the First Wave of the Internet, and identifies key criteria for the success of these firms as being their people, products, platforms, and partnerships, along with a focus on influencing policy and persevering.

The Second Wave of the Internet—according to Case—took place from about 2000 to 2015, and was comprised of companies like Facebook, Google, Snapchat, Amazon, eBay, LinkedIn, and Twitter. In this period, the so-called app economy emerged, and firms didn't need to focus nearly as much effort on partnerships and influencing policy to succeed. Applications for desktop and laptop computers, smartphones, and tablets multiplied, while Google and Facebook (Internet search and social networking) established their dominance essentially on their own. In 2008, Apple began marketing their slogan "There's an App for That", and during this period tens of billions of mobile apps were downloaded.

Case says that we're now in the Third Wave of the Internet, where it is once again necessary for startups and other companies to partner with industry incumbents, work to effect necessary policy changes (for innovation and new business practices to take hold in the marketplace), and persevere to succeed and, in some cases, disrupt sectors like healthcare, education, transportation, energy, and food. According to Case, this next technological revolution will transform the economy and the way we live our lives.

When it comes to disrupting healthcare, however, Vinod Khosla—a venture capitalist and cofounder of Sun Microsystems (one of the First Wave companies identified by Case)—has a different perspective. In a 2012 op-ed in Fortune, Khosla writes that: "Innovation seldom happens from the inside because existing incentives are usually set up to discourage disruption. Pharma companies push marginally different drugs instead of potentially better generic solutions because they want you to be a drug subscriber and generate recurring revenue for as long as possible. Medical device manufacturers don't want to cannibalize sales of their expensive equipment by providing cheaper, more accessible monitoring devices. The traditional players will lobby/goad/pay/intimidate doctors and regulators to reject innovation. Expecting the medical establishment to do anything different is expecting them to reduce their own profits. Granted, these are generalizations and there are many great and ethical doctors and organizations." However, as Khosla points out, disruption will still occur via exogenous innovations: "It doesn't matter if the establishment tries to do this or not, because it will happen regardless. And it may start at the periphery."

In reference to one of these innovations— artificial intelligence (AI)—Khosla predicts that: "Technology will reinvent healthcare as we know it. It is inevitable that, in the future, the majority of physicians' diagnostic, prescription and monitoring, which over time may approach 80-percent of total doctors'/internists' time spent on medicine, will be replaced by smart hardware, software, and testing. This is not to say 80-percent of physicians will be replaced, but rather 80-percent of what they currently do might be replaced so the roles doctors/internists play will likely be different and focused on the human aspects of medical practice such as empathy and ethical choices."

Regarding the potential for AI, automation, and robots (all in the same category) to reduce employment, a recent report from International Data Corporation (IDC) released by Salesforce confirms Khosla's comments. Contrary to what's indicated in many news stories, the report estimates that AI will actually produce a net gain of about 800,000 jobs—up to a potential 2 million new jobs—by 2021. According to the report: "The forecast embodies an assumption that AI will lead to net-positive financial benefits, which will drive job growth. Some roles may be eliminated, and others will be created or enhanced, not unlike the change in jobs in IT departments during the advent of the cloud."

It bears noting that Khosla backs up his statements on the growth potential of AI and other digital health innovations in healthcare and on the periphery with his wallet. As the founder of Khosla Ventures, a venture capital investment firm, he is focused on assisting entrepreneurs to build impactful new energy and technology companies. As of 2016, according to my count, Khosla Ventures is the all-time most prolific private equity investor in digital health, making a total of 40 deals from 2012 through September 2017.

Another perspective on the potential for disruption of established industries comes from Evgeny Morozov, author of 'The Net Delusion: The Dark Side of Internet Freedom', and 'To Save Everything, Click Here:

The Folly of Technological Solutionism.' In a 2016 op-ed, 'Silicon Valley was going to disrupt capitalism. Now it's just enhancing it,' Morozov writes: "The tech giants thought they would beat old businesses, but the health and finance industries are using data troves to become more, not less, resilient." Morozov points out that partnerships (of the variety described by Case) are not actually poised to transform established industries like healthcare. He uses two examples to illustrate how technology companies are not adversaries driving disruption of established business models, but instead coexisting with incumbents via partnerships.

The perspectives of Christensen, Case, Khosla, and Morozov all have their own merits and exceptions, particularly in reference to digital health. In this regard, I've identified four key digital health strategies of note being pursued by companies and organizations: enhancement, multifaceted, adjacent, and disruption. In addition, I've identified a few unique approaches being pursued by healthcare providers. It's important to note that these methods and approaches are valid and will result in benefits to human health.

Enhancement

The first company exemplifying one of the four noteworthy digital health strategies is Alphabet, one of the Silicon Valley tech giants mentioned by Evgeny Morozov. Alphabet is a holding company for a variety of subsidiaries: Calico, DeepMind, Google, Google Fiber, Jigsaw, Nest Labs, Sidewalk Labs, Verily, Waymo, and X. This heritage—and the relationships between the subsidiaries—means that they typically have strong capabilities in data gathering, handling, and analysis.

Some of the strategies being pursued by Alphabet's subsidiaries include standalone efforts and noteworthy partnerships and joint ventures with incumbent players in healthcare:

- DeepMind: The AI-focused company has a health unit focused on "Helping clinicians get patients from test to treatment, faster." The subsidiary recently experienced a data-sharing consent and privacy controversy after the Royal Free NHS Trust—which operates three hospitals within the UK's National Health Service (NHS)—shared 1.6 million patient medical records with DeepMind, apparently without either of the two entities informing or asking for consent from the patients themselves.
- Verily Life Sciences describes itself as being "at the intersection of technology, data science, and healthcare. Our mission is to make the world's health data useful so that people enjoy healthier lives." The company has formed several noteworthy partnerships and joint ventures:
  - Partnered with Sanofi to form Onduo, a joint venture focused on helping people with diabetes live full, healthy lives by developing comprehensive solutions that combine devices, software, medicine, and professional care to enable simple and intelligent disease management.

- o Partnered with Johnson & Johnson's Ethicon unit to form Verb Surgical, a joint venture building a digital surgery platform that combines robotics, advanced visualization, instrumentation, data analytics and connectivity.
- o Partnered with GlaxoSmithKline (GSK) to form Galvani Bioelectronics, a joint venture focused on developing bioelectronic medicines. 'Bioelectronic medicine' uses tiny implantable devices to change precise electrical signals in nerves to treat a range of debilitating chronic diseases.
- o Partnering with Novartis' Alcon unit to develop smart ocular devices, including a glucose-sensing lens for continuous monitoring of glucose levels, and a contact lens for people with presbyopia (age-related farsightedness).
- o Partnering with Dexcom to develop miniaturized continuous glucose monitors to help people with Type 2 diabetes manage the condition.
- o Partnering with Biogen and Brigham and Women's Hospital to understand why multiple sclerosis (MS) progresses so differently among diagnosed individuals and to glean insights that could inform new therapies and improve care for all MS patients.

- Partnering with 3M Health Information Systems (HIS) to develop a technology platform focused on delivering population health measurement tools and services. The platform will analyze population-level health data sets with the goal of helping hospitals surface meaningful information that can be used to improve healthcare quality and reduce costs. It will combine 3M's health data coding, classification, and risk-stratification tools with Verily's data analytics, software tools, and algorithms.

- Calico: Partnering with Abbvie on the development of new medicines focused on aging and age-related diseases, including neurodegeneration and cancer.

- Google: Primarily focused on web-based search and display advertising tools, desktop systems, consumer content, enterprise solutions, commerce, and hardware products.

  - More than 2 billion mobile devices use the company's Android mobile operating system. However, the majority of these devices are manufactured by other companies.

  - The company reportedly wants to leverage its big data analytics capability to take over the payer function of the Centers of Medicare & Medicaid Services (CMS). CMS is part of the U.S. Department of Health and Human

Services (HHS) and administers Medicare, Medicaid, the Children's Health Insurance Program (CHIP), and the Health Insurance Marketplace.

There are other Alphabet subsidiaries engaged in efforts relevant to digital health, including X's Project Loon, which received approval from the Federal Communications Commission (FCC) to deploy its network of high altitude balloons to Puerto Rico in an effort to restore cellular and Internet communications in the aftermath of Hurricane Maria.

Another subsidiary—Sidewalk Labs—is redeveloping up to 800 acres of waterfront in Toronto, Canada to create a smart city that leverages technology to improve people's lives. The planned urban environment will include a multitude of embedded sensors of all types, which will gather a constant stream of data regarding pedestrian and vehicle traffic, noise levels, air quality, energy usage, and waste output. Cameras will also record how people interact with such things as public furniture in green spaces and whether residents use popup clinics during flu season.

The work being done by Alphabet, its subsidiaries, and partners is incredibly important in terms of advancing the field of medicine, treating and curing diseases, and improving human health and wellbeing. From a business perspective, however, these are mostly not indicative of potential disruption of healthcare systems, the medical device, or the pharmaceutical industries—either within them or at the peripheries.

Multifaceted

Apple—which has a digital platform of more than 1 billion mobile devices using its iOS operating system—is uniquely positioned in digital health. The tech giant is best known for its iPhone, iPad, and Apple Watch products. It also makes AirPods, which are worn in the ear and contain speakers, microphones, voice and motion accelerometers, optical sensors, and an onboard computer with wireless functionality. Recent patents by the company point to the possibility of future AirPods containing biometric sensors for use in measuring heart rate; blood oxygen (VO2) levels; galvanic skin response (GSR) (to determine stress levels); electrocardiogram (EKG) and impedance cardiography (ICG) (for measuring heart electrical activity); and a temperature sensor (for use as a thermometer).

At the company's big product launch event in September 2017, it announced that the third version of the Watch will, as rumored, come with LTE (mobile phone cellular network) capability onboard, thus untethering the device from the iPhone as its link to the Internet. This improved functionality and mobility is important for improving the available features and user interface for health and medical applications. Other noteworthy new features include activity coaching, a swimming app, and a gym equipment connection function (for obtaining workout data from wireless-enabled gym equipment). There's also an updated heart rate monitor, which will measure and track resting heart rate, heart rhythm, recovery heart rate, and provide a notification if it detects an elevated heart rate when you're not active.

The improved heart monitoring capabilities are fascinating, as Apple reportedly wants the Watch to be able to detect atrial fibrillation (AFib), the most common type of heart arrhythmia. AFib is characterized by the heart beating too slowly, too fast, or in an irregular way. Some people with AFib don't have any symptoms or know they have it, as it often goes undiagnosed. AFib is a major population health problem, with the CDC estimating that from 2.7 to 6.1 million in the U.S. have it. The condition accounts for 50,000 hospitalizations each year and contributes to an estimated 130,000 deaths. Healthcare costs for AFib are $6 billion per year in the U.S. and costs for people who have AFib are nearly $9,000 higher per year than for people who don't have it.

Apple also has a suite of dedicated digital health apps and development platforms: the 'Health' app for consumers comes native to all iPhones; 'HealthKit', which is used by health & fitness app developers to collate and share data; 'CareKit', which is for healthcare and medical app developers; and 'ResearchKit', which is for clinical and medical researchers.

In addition to its in-house innovation efforts, Apple is also pursuing partnerships and mergers and acquisitions (M&A) in the following notable areas:

- Health Insurance – Aetna is partnering with Apple to develop health initiatives and will reportedly provide the Apple Watch for free—or at a reduced-cost—to its 23 million health insurance customers. Aetna is also giving the Apple Watch to its 50,000 employees.

- Independent Aging – In partnership with IBM and Japan Post (the largest health insurance company in Japan), Apple is providing millions of senior citizens with iPads containing apps focused on health, family, and community engagement. These include a medication reminder app and the FaceTime video app, which can be used to communicate with family members and non-medical service providers.

- Connected Transportation – Apple invested $1 billion in Didi, aka the Uber of China. Apple is also an indirect investor in Uber, due to Didi's $1 billion investment in the company. Connected transportation and autonomous vehicles present enormous opportunities for human health (more on that in a later section).

- Sleep – Apple recently acquired Beddit, a startup focused on sleep tracking and improvement. The company's primary device is a thin strip of sensors (placed across a user's bed) that gathers and analyzes sleep time, sleep efficiency, heart rate, respiration, temperature, movement, snoring, room temperature, and room humidity. In October 2017, the Beddit Sleep Monitor was listed as sold out in Apple's online store. However, it's likely that the product or technology will reemerge as a part of a future Apple-branded sleep monitoring, management, and improvement system.

- Electronic Health Records (EHR) – Epic Systems— a major provider of EHRs to hospitals and large medical groups—is integrating consumer-generated health data (gathered from a wide range of consumer devices and apps) collected in Apple's HealthKit and then ported into the company's MyChart app. In turn, Epic's 170 million patients can use HealthKit through the MyChart app, which also contains elements of their own patient record.
- Personal Health Records (PHR) – In 2016, Apple acquired Gliimpse, a startup that offered a secure platform for consumers to collect, manage, and share their own medical records and health information. It's also been reported that Apple is partnering with another startup, Health Gorilla, to add a patient's medical diagnostic testing results onto their iPhone.

As part of its digital health strategy, Apple has reportedly created its own fitness lab. Jay Blahnik, Apple's director of fitness for health technologies, recently stated that over the past five years, the company's fitness lab has collected more data on activity and exercise than any other human performance study in history. To date, he says, there have been over 10,000 unique participants (contrast this with a typical medical clinical trial of less than 100 enrollees), who have completed 33,000 sessions and generated more than 66,000 hours of data. Apple employees exercise in group classes, on rowing machines, treadmills, cable machines, and even swim in an endless pool, all while 13 exercise physiologists and 29 nurses and medics monitor data obtained from the Apple Watch, metabolic carts, ECGs, and a mask that tracks calorie burn, oxygen consumption, and VO2 max. Apple's fitness lab also has rooms with microclimates that simulate Arctic conditions (subfreezing) and desert heat (above 100°F / 37.8°C).

Augmented reality (AR) has emerged as a major focus for Apple, which has just released its ARKit, a tool intended to enable developers to build AR applications for the iPhone and iPad. In a recent interview, Apple CEO Tim Cook explained how AR will change our lives: "Think back to 2008, when the App Store went live. There was the initial round of apps and people looked at them and said, 'this is not anything, mobile apps are not going to take off'. And then, step by step, things start to move. And it is sort of a curve, it was just exponential—and now you couldn't imagine your life without apps. Your health is on one app, your financials, your shopping, your news, your entertainment—it's everything. AR is like that. It will be that dramatic." And more recently, Cook stated: "We believe AR is going to change the way we use technology forever. Virtual models for everything you can imagine, from the human body to the solar system."

Technology critic David Pogue conducted a video review of seven of the first iPhone AR apps and stated that: "For my money, augmented reality (AR) is the bigger deal (versus virtual reality (VR)). That's where you can still see the real world, but the computer superimposes graphics on it. As you look around, the sizes, angles, and distances of the simulated objects smoothly change in real time as though they really exist. Pokémon Go is an AR app. So is Snapchat when it adds goofy glasses and antennae to your live image." One of the examples Pogue features in his review is the Ikea Place app, which lets users see how Ikea furniture will fit in their actual home or office.

Tim Cook has also shared information on his rationale for pursuing digital health as a business opportunity: "We've gotten into the health arena and we started looking at wellness, that took us to pulling a string to thinking about research, pulling that string a little further took us to some patient-care stuff, and that pulled a string that's taking us into some other stuff. When you look at most of the solutions—whether it's devices, or things coming up out of Big Pharma—first and foremost, they are done to get the reimbursement (from an insurance provider), not thinking about what helps the patient. So, if you don't care about reimbursement—which we have the privilege of doing— that may even make the smartphone market look small." Cook has also stated that: "We're extremely interested in this area. And, yes, it is a business opportunity. If you look at it, medical health activity is the largest or second-largest component of the economy, depending on which country in the world you're dealing with."

When looking at Apple's overarching digital health strategy and related bets on innovative new products and services, the history of the company under Steve Jobs is worth considering. As well-known Apple analyst and tech critic Rene Ritchie observed: "With one slide Steve Jobs took Apple's most successful product, iPod, and rendered it down to an app on (the then unproven) iPhone." Ritchie adds that: "Not mistaking their products for their businesses is what let Apple makes giant leaps in the past."

Entering new markets via digital health products and series makes business sense for Apple, as the revenue growth opportunities are enormous. According to Rick Tetzeli, editor-at-large with Fast Company: "Annual global health spending is more than $9 trillion. And while Apple may not currently dominate any of these arenas, remember that analysts once thought Apple would have a hit on its hands if it could garner 1% of the mobile phone business. One percent of $9 trillion is $90 billion. Even Apple might call that a pretty good business."

For Apple—with the diversified markets it's entering—the aggregate revenue growth opportunity is significantly larger than that provided by the healthcare segment alone. In considering these opportunities (refer to my chart 'Market Opportunities for Digital Health'), if Apple can capture 1% of $43 trillion, that equates to an additional $430 billion in revenue, or nearly $200 billion more than its 2015 revenue of $234 billion. Moreover, it's clear that Apple is looking to take a big chunk out of the augmented reality (AR) and virtual reality (VR) markets, which could reach $182 billion by 2025.

Apple's strategy of leveraging its digital customer interface places it directly in the value chain between consumers and their health, wellness, healthcare providers, and employers. In parallel and overlapping fashion, Apple is also building interfaces and integrating into the ecosystem of healthcare stakeholders, including providers, insurers, and electronic health records (EHR) system suppliers. Moreover, Apple is working with medical and clinical researchers. The company's sweeping strategy is enabled by in-house solutions, M&A, and partnerships, providing it with a mix of disruptive and enhancement business opportunities. As such, Apple is a prime example of what I call a multifaceted digital health strategy.

Adjacent

Over the past few years, Under Armour (UA)—a performance footwear, apparel, and equipment company—has entered digital health in a major way. Between 2013 and 2015, the company acquired three health and fitness apps—MapMyFitness, MyFitnessPal, and Endomondo—for a total cost of more than $700 million. The apps integrate with UA's existing UA Record app and devices (plus hundreds of third-party devices), collectively forming the company's health and fitness platform named 'Under Armour Connected Fitness'. UA claims that this platform—an example of a digital customer interface—has more than 200 million registered users and that more than 90% of them have specific health goals.

The digital health devices sold by UA include a fitness- and sleep-tracking wristband, a chest-worn heart rate monitor, wireless heart rate monitoring headphones, and a smart scale. Moreover, it sells 'Record Equipped' running shoes, which feature a built-in chip that tracks and reports running metrics aimed at helping improve a runner's performance. After 400 miles the shoes will also notify users that it's time to buy a new pair.

UA is also partnering with Johns Hopkins Medicine in a collaboration designed to help athletes maintain and improve health, wellness, and recovery. Noteworthy is that a team of sleep experts—led by Dr. Alan Schwartz, director of the Sleep Disorders Center at Johns Hopkins Bayview Medical Center—is working with UA on a multiphase research study that includes guidance on an algorithm related to sleep quality, patterns, and behaviors. Following an 18-month study involving NFL football player Tom Brady—who attributes part of his career success to getting enough sleep for optimal recovery—UA created its TB12 far infrared bioceramic-printed sleep garment. According to UA's chief technology officer, Paul Fipps, the athlete recovery sleepwear, wearable sleep tracker, and companion app system "lets people track their sleep so they can take steps to improve the quality of their sleep. This, in turn, will allow them to recover faster and perform better. The experience is about the physical and the digital, not just one or the other."

While sleep is a critical component of recovery for athletes, it's also vital to our overall health, with the Centers for Disease Control (CDC) even stating that insufficient sleep is a public health problem. Sleep insufficiency is linked to motor vehicle crashes, industrial disasters, and medical and other occupational errors. Persons experiencing sleep insufficiency are also more likely to suffer from chronic diseases such as hypertension, diabetes, depression, obesity, as well as from cancer, which is not always a one-time event and can sometimes be treated like a chronic disease. They also have reduced quality of life and productivity and increased mortality risk. While sleep insufficiency can be caused by a range of societal factors—such as round-the-clock access to technology and work schedules—sleep disorders such as insomnia and obstructive sleep apnea also play a role. In the U.S., there are an estimated 50-70 million adults who have a sleep or wakefulness disorder.

With UA's focus on health, fitness, nutrition, recovery, and sleep, and a digital health platform of more than 200 million highly-motivated users, it's justifiable that company CEO, Kevin Plank, envisions that Under Armour Connected Fitness will "fundamentally affect global health." In a recent interview, Plank also highlighted a few glaring blind spots in the healthcare status quo: "The most important asset anyone has is health, but why is it that we know the least about it? When I ask how many days were you sick last year, why don't you know? You could have $400 in a checking account and the bank would send reams of data. But if I ask, "How's your health?" You'll say, "I don't know. I feel pretty good; I was at the doctor 18 months ago." And UA is apparently seeking to address this gap, at least in part: "Our consumer wants us to have more information about them, and we need to give them something back. When they give us data and tell us this about themselves, how are we using that to inform, to make their lives easier and better?"

Similar to the key elements allowing Google to disrupt the newspaper industry, UA's Connected Fitness platform is an example of a digital customer interface comprised of high-intent users. However, while UA also sells advertising on its platform, unlike Google, the sales generated on its digital efforts accounted for just a small fraction of 2015 revenue: $53 million out of a total $4 billion in sales. Still, it represents a growth area for the company, as digital sales were up 178% from the prior year. Interestingly, Plank sees the company's digital transformation as fundamental to its overarching business transformation efforts.

Since UA is not a healthcare company, but has a platform with a large user base of consumers—not patients, necessarily—I classify it as operating adjacent to healthcare. Or, paraphrasing Khosla: UA's efforts are an example of disruption at the periphery of healthcare.

Disruption

As I found when looking at the most-downloaded health and fitness apps in January 2017, a menstrual cycle tracking app named Period Tracker Lite was in the top eight. There are more than 1,000 apps in the app stores intended to help women track their menstrual cycles, conceive, or avoid pregnancy. This represents an important category of digital health empowering women's health and wellbeing.

In 2017, one such app—Natural Cycles—became the first app to be approved as a contraceptive and fertility-tracking solution in the European Union. The system works by analyzing changes in a woman's body temperature (which she measures herself using a highly accurate basal body thermometer) and providing information that helps her more closely monitor cycle trends. In a major clinical study of more than 4,000 women, Natural Cycles was 93% effective in preventing pregnancy. This compares to the pill, which has an effectiveness rate of 99.7% when used perfectly. However, in actual use, the effectiveness rate of the pill drops below that of Natural Cycles, to around 92%.

The Natural Cycles app is an example of disruption because it is more effective than a drug and effectively replaces it, or at least offers an alternative. Granted, there are health benefits for women who take the pill, including reducing acne, making periods regular, and easing menstrual cramps. According to Planned Parenthood, the combination pill can also reduce or help prevent: bone thinning; cysts in the breasts and ovaries; endometrial and ovarian cancers; serious infections in the ovaries, fallopian tubes, and uterus; iron deficiency (anemia); and premenstrual syndrome (PMS). But, like many drugs, there are also potential disadvantages and negative side effects. For instance, with the pill and combinations pills, the hormones contained in them can change a woman's level of sexual desire and there may also be bleeding between periods, sore breasts, and nausea.

Natural Cycles is an illustration of a digital health innovation occurring outside an established industry (pharmaceuticals) and directly disrupting it by targeting and seeking to replace an existing product (a pharmaceutical drug). Moreover, since the app can also be used to help women conceive, it joins several other digital health solutions entering the fertility services market, which is projected to exceed $21 billion by 2020. While Natural Cycles alone is unlikely to reach the scale and impact that Google had in disrupting an industry, it represents a fascinating category of digital health that combines devices, sensors, consumers, and apps to create a new mode of healthcare. Significantly, it also provides women more choice in how they manage their own health.

Further indication of the potential for digital health to disrupt the pharmaceutical industry's traditional 'drug-only' model occurred in October 2017, when four digital health companies—Akili Interactive, Propeller Health, Voluntis, and WellDoc—joined forces to create a new organization called the Digital Therapeutics Alliance (DTA). The organization is focused on enhancing patient outcomes through assessing the value and impact of digital therapeutics (DTx) solutions in clinical practice, constructing industry and regulatory frameworks, and encouraging data-driven integration, and utilization of DTx solutions across the healthcare industry. I included another DTx company—Pear Therapeutics—in the list of recent FDA digital health approvals.

Healthcare

Unlike most countries around the world, the delivery of healthcare in the United States is a hodgepodge of four different systems: the Beveridge Model, the Bismarck Model, the National Health Insurance Model, and the Out-of-Pocket Model. While I won't go into all of these in detail, PBS provides a useful explainer from T. R. Reid's book, 'The Healing of America: A Global Quest for Better, Cheaper, and Fairer Health Care'.

What's noteworthy is that the CDC's 2016 National Health Interview Survey indicated that 65% of people in the U.S. under the age of 65 have private insurance—which falls within the 'Out-of-Pocket Model' healthcare system. This is characterized by people having private health insurance, often offered through employers or other organizations. It can also be purchased by individuals, for example through the Patient Protection and Affordable Care Act (ACA), also known as Obamacare.

According to the Commonwealth Fund, "Prior to the passage of the Affordable Care Act, the individual insurance market was a notoriously difficult place for consumers without employer-based health benefits to purchase insurance. It also was challenging for insurers to sell insurance without incurring large losses. As a result, insurers went to great lengths to exclude people with even mild health problems. In 2010, the Commonwealth Fund Biennial Health Insurance Survey found that more than one-third of people who tried to purchase health insurance in the individual market in the previous three years—an estimated 9 million people—had been turned down, charged a higher price, or had a condition excluded from their health plan. By January 2016, near the end of the ACA's fourth open-enrollment period, things had changed. The size of the individual market has nearly doubled since 2010."

Many healthcare provider systems in the United States must work with payers—including private health insurance companies and government health insurers (like Medicare and Medicaid)—to be reimbursed for the services they provide to patients. This model inherently discourages certain types of innovations and cost savings offered by digital health. Essentially, there is little incentive for providers to lower costs since the result would be decreased revenue from payers.

As Khosla eloquently stated, "Innovation seldom happens from the inside because existing incentives are usually set up to discourage disruption." Apple's Cook echoes the same point: "When you look at most of the solutions, whether it's devices, or things coming up out of Big Pharma, first and foremost, they are done to get the reimbursement (from an insurance provider)."

In the U.S., there are a couple of notable exceptions to the more prevalent healthcare system model. The incentives in these systems offer a significantly more favorable environment for digital health innovation to occur.

The Veterans Health Administration (VHA)—part of the U.S. Department of Veterans Affairs (VA)—is the largest integrated healthcare system in the United States, providing care to more than 9 million enrolled veterans each year. Comprised of 1,243 health care facilities—including 170 medical centers and 1,063 outpatient sites of care—the VHA is both a provider and a payer. This structure provides internal incentives to reduce costs overall while also improving the quality of care. Consequently, the VHA has been a pioneer in digital health innovation, particularly in telehealth.

In 2013, more than 600,000 VHA patients received some element of their healthcare via telehealth, with the total for all telehealth episodes of care equaling 1.7 million. Note that telehealth—which encompasses telemedicine—is a technology-enabled means of changing the location where healthcare services are routinely provided. This is particularly vital for serving rural populations and patients who may have other difficulties getting to healthcare facilities.

According to Adam Darkins, MD, who served as chief consultant at the VA and architect of its telehealth programs from 2003 to 2014: "Telehealth in VA is the forerunner of a wider vision, one in which the relationship between patients and the healthcare system will dramatically change with the full realization of the connected patient. The high levels of patient satisfaction with telehealth and positive clinical outcome attest to this direction being the right one."

The second notable example of a healthcare provider system offering greater opportunities for digital health to thrive is Kaiser Permanente (KP). With over 11 million members, California-based KP is one of the nation's largest not-for-profit health insurance and healthcare providers. Unlike many other healthcare systems, it is an integrated managed care consortium consisting of three separate entities: a health plan (that bears insurance risk), medical groups of physicians, and a hospital system. According to a report by the Brookings Institution, KP's financial incentive is to provide high quality, affordable care, and management of population health rather than focusing on generating a high volume of compensable services.

According to KP's website, they have "an integrated structure that allows the health plan, the hospital and the physicians and medical group to work together in a coordinated fashion for the benefit of the patient. This level of integration, supported by sophisticated information technology, means that the patient, along with her/his appropriate medical information, can move smoothly from the clinic to the hospital or from primary care to specialty care." This highlights an issue of health data interoperability, which separate healthcare systems encounter when patients move between them.

KP goes on to the highlight the importance and return on investment (ROI) of disease prevention and population health efforts, which are typically not part of other healthcare systems due to challenges around obtaining reimbursement for these types of services: "There are many other important features of the Kaiser Permanente system. We have an intense focus on prevention, health education and care management. Using these programs, we have systematically reduced the death rate from cardiovascular disease and colon cancer significantly below the California average. Our goal is to keep people healthy so that they can live long and thrive!"

Regarding Kaiser Permanente's digital health strategy, Bernard J. Tyson, Chairman & CEO, states that: "The doctor's office of the future will be designed with the patient in mind and as much focused on keeping them healthy as treating them when they are sick." Tyson adds that: "Technology is key to making care more connected, convenient and accessible. Telemedicine will offer consumers care at the touch of a button. Better interoperability of electronic health records across the country will ensure we're providing everyone with the coordinated care that's necessary for us to succeed. That doesn't mean more technology always means better care, it means we need to understand how technology can improve the care our wonderful nurses and physicians already provide. If I were designing our system from scratch I would design it around technology, not buildings."

The results of KP's digital health and related efforts to improve the delivery, quality, and outcomes of healthcare are impressive. Between 2008 and 2014, heart attack rates fell 23% among nearly 4 million KP members in Northern California. And in Donald Jones' video from 2009 (as I recounted in my introduction, this is the video that first inspired my efforts in digital health) he indicates that KP research, at that time, indicated that that more than 50% of primary healthcare could be done virtually (via telehealth). Fast forward to 2016, and Tyson, speaking at Salesforce's annual Dreamforce conference in San Francisco, stated that: "For the first time, last year (2015), we had over 110 million interactions between our physicians and our members." Tyson added that 52% of these interactions were done via smartphone, videoconferencing, kiosks, and other technology tools.

Telehealth

Telehealth is a form of digital health that provides a wide range of benefits, including greater convenience and timeliness of care for patients, improved access to nurses, doctors, and specialists, and cost-savings to healthcare providers.

The Health Resources and Services Administration (HRSA)—part of the U.S. Department of

Health and Human Services (HHS)—broadly defines telehealth as the use of electronic information and telecommunications technologies to support and promote long-distance clinical healthcare, patient and professional health-related education, public health, and health administration. Technologies used for this purpose include videoconferencing, the Internet, store-and-forward imaging, streaming media, and terrestrial and wireless communications.

Some of the biggest dedicated telehealth providers and platforms in the U.S. are American Well, MDLIVE, Doctor on Demand, and Teladoc. In addition to direct-to-consumer (DTC) business models, healthcare systems will often contract with these companies—which supply the technology and the contracted doctors and therapists—or they will use their own medical staff to provide virtual/telehealth medical visits.

Founded in 2009, MDLIVE was one of the first dedicated telehealth providers. The company's service covers more than 20 million people, a number expected to reach 22 million by the end of 2017. It also offers small employers in the U.S. (a market size of approximately 28 million businesses) health and wellness packages for their employees. The company recently partnered with DermatologistOnCall to offers virtual dermatology visits. And, with a network of more than 1,300 mental health professionals, it recently became the first telehealth provider to offer psychiatric services in all 50 states.

There is a critical need for mental health services in the U.S., as approximately 20% of the population experiences mental illness each year according to data compiled by the National Alliance on Mental Illness (NAMI). MDLIVE's CEO, Scott Decker, sees the virtual psychiatry market as tremendously untapped and states that: "It could be as big as our core business over time, and it probably fits our model even better than a basic physician office visit. A virtual visit can take away the stigma that has been associated with behavior health issues."

In China, telehealth is also gaining in popularity. Ping An Haoyisheng—aka Ping An Good Doctor—was founded in 2015 by Ping An Insurance. The service provides subscribers with 24/7 access to consultations with medical specialists, who can provide a quick diagnosis, treatment, drug prescriptions, and book additional appointments. With over 77 million registered users, Ping An claims to deliver more than 250,000 consultations each day provided by over 1,000 full-time medical professionals and an additional network of 50,000 doctors. The company expects to grow to 500 million users by 2019.

Also in China, search engine giant Baidu is providing an AI-powered conversational chatbot for use by patients and doctors. Melody, as 'she' is known, integrates with the Baidu Doctor app and provides a form of virtual triage by gathering relevant medical information from patients and providing it to their doctors. Interestingly, Melody also suggests possible treatment options directly to the doctor. This is known as clinical decision support (CDS). Doctors can choose to communicate these AI-generated recommendations directly to their patients, or develop their own diagnoses and treatment recommendations. According to Andrew

Ng, Baidu's chief scientist: "Melody is designed to help both doctors and patients. By focusing on the medical assistant space, we've built a conversational bot that can give highly-customized and situation-appropriate responses to a patient's query. As Melody has more conversations, it will learn and keep getting better. This is just the start of a much larger AI-driven transformation of the healthcare industry."

In pointing out how the Melody AI system learns, Ng highlights what is called machine learning. This is the ability of a computer to learn without being explicitly programmed. I include another example of this in the Imaging section.

Opportunities

Digital health is already impacting our health, healthcare, how we live our lives, and many aspects of society. Moving forward, these impacts will continue to multiply and grow in force. The following are a few key areas where the transformational potential and opportunities are particularly noteworthy.

Chronic Disease

According to the U.S. Centers for Disease Control (CDC), chronic diseases account for 86% of annual healthcare expenditures. Since the U.S. healthcare system is primarily focused on treating people when they become sick—versus preventing sickness and disease—it should come as no surprise that many digital health companies and other entities are filling this gap by focusing—either directly or indirectly—on combating chronic diseases. As previously discussed, the economic burdens of healthcare costs are placed on all stakeholders. This incentivizes cost-cutting via digital health innovation and other means, thereby creating business opportunities.

The most common and costly chronic diseases include heart disease (aka cardiovascular disease), certain types of cancer, type 2 diabetes, and obesity. Between 2015 and 2016, nearly 40% of U.S. adults and nearly 19% of youths were classified as obese. Also, the number of obese children and adolescents (aged 5-19 years) worldwide has increased tenfold in the past four decades, growing from 11 million in 1975 to 124 million in 2016.

Half of all American adults have at least one chronic condition, with around 33% having multiple chronic conditions, aka comorbities. While genetic factors can contribute to the risk of chronic disease, they (chronic diseases) are typically preventable. The worst disease risk-increasing behaviors include: lack of exercise, physical inactivity, poor diet and nutrition, tobacco use and secondhand smoke, and drinking too much alcohol. Combined, these unhealthy lifestyle choices cause much of the illness, suffering, and early death related to chronic diseases and conditions. According to the World Health Organization (WHO), cardiovascular disease (CVD) is the number one cause of death globally. An estimated 17.7 million people died from CVDs in 2015, which amounts to 31% of all global deaths.

In 2015, 50% of U.S. adults did not meet recommendations for aerobic physical activity. This is significant, because physical activity reduces the risks of cardiovascular disease and diabetes beyond that produced by weight reduction alone. Physical activity provides a variety of health benefits by helping to: maintain weight; reduce high blood pressure; and reduce the risk for type 2 diabetes, heart attack, stroke, and several forms of cancer. Physical activity also helps reduce arthritis pain and associated disability, the risk for osteoporosis and falls, and even symptoms of depression and anxiety. Moreover, studies have shown that the risk of early death is as low for those who meet recommended activity targets in one or two sessions per week as it is for daily exercisers. In other words, 'weekend warriors', or people who may not exercise as consistently during a work week, still derive important benefits from exercising just a couple of days each week.

Excessive sedentary time is common in Western societies. In 2014, 83 million people in the United States lived a sedentary lifestyle, meaning they spent most of their time during the day sitting, or performed little to no physical activity. A recent study funded by the National Institutes of Health (NIH) concluded that being sedentary for long periods of time—particularly in prolonged, uninterrupted bouts—is associated with all-cause mortality. In other words: 'sitting around all day' leads to an increased risk of all types of death. In fact, the World Health Organization states that physical inactivity is the fourth leading risk factor for mortality, causing an estimated 3.2 million deaths globally each year.

Investigators who conducted a meta-analysis of studies on physical inactivity concluded that prolonged sitting of 8-12 hours per day increases the risk of developing type 2 diabetes by 90%. Even if you exercise, sitting too much during the day will still raise your risk of disability, heart disease, obesity, and certain types of cancer. For every two hours spent sitting in front of a TV or computer, an average person will increase their cancer risk by 66%. For colon cancer, the risk increases 24%, for endometrial cancer the risk goes up 32%, and for lung cancer the risk is 21% greater.

Physical inactivity also accelerates the aging process. A study found that retired persons who maintained a sedentary position for ten hours or more per day—and who did less than 40 minutes of moderate physical activity—had the bodies of people eight years older. This was determined by looking at the lengths of their telomeres, the tiny caps found on the ends of strands of DNA. These protect chromosomes and shorter lengths—like those observed in the study participants—are associated with faster aging, according to researchers.

When it comes to digital health and physical activity, most people naturally think of fitness apps and wearable tech devices like the Fitbit and Apple Watch. While these tools can't force people to be more physically active, they can serve as a means of tracking physical activity and providing reminders and nudges to motivate activity.

For example, in addition to activity rings—which can serve to motivate people to move around and exercise a certain amount per day in order to complete the circles—the Apple Watch has a notification feature that prods users to get up and move (or at least stand up) after 50 minutes of inactivity. Apple CEO Tim Cook has stated that, when wearing the device, executives at his company will jump up at the same time during meetings. And while Cook has stated that: "It took a while to get used to, but it's actually really good. A lot of doctors believe sitting is the new cancer", it's more likely that what he meant to say was: 'sitting is the new smoking'.

Even Facebook provides subtle nudges, for example by posting a note in a person's timeline describing the weather outside and what attire to wear.

For many people, just thinking about being outside can be a motivator to do just that.

As anyone who has tried to exercise more—or simply maintain a certain level of physical activity—knows, behavior change can be challenging. And even if digital nudges are insufficiently motivating, or apps and devices are abandoned, the important thing is that we maintain healthy levels of physical activity. While not necessary, digital tools can help to educate and motivate us—including via social networks, where we motivate and challenge one another. There's no one-size-fits-all approach. I use very simple digital tools for my chosen sport of surfing. This includes a digital watch with pre-programmed ocean tides and an app on my smartphone and computer. They're not necessary, but they are important aids that foster increased enjoyment of my sport and frequency, thereby producing health benefits, particularly in helping to reduce my risk of chronic diseases.

Some other examples of digital tools facilitating physical activity include apps like ClassPass and Mindbody, which help people find individual and group fitness and yoga classes, as well as other wellness services. There are also a wide variety of apps for tracking physical activity and sporting endeavors—some with virtual coaching features—that can be found in the Apple iTunes and Google Play app stores.

There are also a few fascinating examples of online fitness coaching and group exercise workouts, including well-known Peloton, which offers live-streaming interactive studio cycling classes. Participating from their home, users riding a stationary bike with a large video screen can see and hear the instructors while also viewing real-time performance metrics, including cadence, resistance, and output, even a leaderboard. All of this contributes to an engaging and competitive workout that motivates people to not only push their performance, but continue using the service.

Another application of digital tools being leveraged to help improve physical workout performance and results comes from Orangetheory Fitness, which offers group personal training classes. By using wearable devices that track heart rate, calories burned, and percentage of effort, users and their trainers can better monitor their heart rate based interval training, which helps them maintain a target zone that both stimulates metabolism and increases energy.

While physical activity and other healthy behaviors are of critical value in reducing disease risk, they are equally important to people who already have one or more chronic conditions. Digital tools inherently afford considerable benefits in this regard, particularly when coupled with human interaction, intervention, and expert coaching.

A noteworthy example of this comes from Twine Health, which provides a health coaching platform that helps patients prevent, monitor, and reverse chronic disease. Counting more than 50 workplace health providers and healthcare delivery system customers, the company's health coaching platform enables users to create their own health action plan within a self-management app. The app is then programmed to send reminders to users to take their medications, plus provide guidance around planned lifestyle changes, including diet and exercise. Trends in medication adherence and progress made—or not made—towards goals are also made available to health coaches, healthcare providers, family, and friends, who provide vital and timely support and encouragement in addition to ongoing refinement of the plan. The overarching goals include improving participants' quality of life, health outcomes, and providing cost savings to all stakeholders.

Again, whether aided by digital tools or not, it's vital to your health that you stay active and pursue other healthy behaviors to reduce your risk of chronic diseases. For people who already have one or more chronic diseases, it's critical that they manage them so that they don't worsen. It's even possible—as I cover in one example—to reverse some chronic diseases. Moreover, since chronic disease is responsible for 86% of all healthcare costs, disease prevention represents a peripheral opportunity—on the part of consumers and patients—to disrupt the healthcare system in much the same way that Google disrupted the newspaper industry: by taking away its primary revenue source.

Genetic Testing

There are more than 1,000 genetic tests in use today. These fall within three main categories: Chromosomal (which looks at whole chromosomes or long lengths of DNA), Molecular (focused on single genes or short lengths of DNA to identify variations or mutations), and Biochemical (examines the amount or activity level of proteins). These tests—which are available through healthcare providers (physicians, nurse practitioners, and genetic counselors) or direct-to-consumer (DTC)—provide actionable information for consumers, patients, and doctors.

In medicine, genetic testing can provide disease diagnosis, help identify the correct drugs and drug dosing (aka pharmacogenomics), and provide insights into disease risks. For consumers, DTC genetic tests (typically advertised via television, in print media, and on the Internet) can provide insights into genealogy (tracing of family lineages and history), as well as health indicators, including caffeine metabolism, certain disease risk levels, and carrier status of inherited conditions (for family planning).

A key point is that many medically-relevant tests for disease risk—like one's genetic risk of Parkinson's disease and late-onset Alzheimer's, for example—can be obtained directly by a consumer without a healthcare provider's permission or order. Companies offering this type of DTC service include 23andMe, Color Genomics, and Counsyl. However, it is important to note that disease risk is not the same as a disease diagnosis, nor is risk indicative of a certitude that someone will get a disease. In other words, DNA is not always destiny. Moreover, it is possible that these tests can return a false positive or false negative. Nonetheless, these types of tests are informative and can guide as well as reinforce the significance of behavioral lifestyle choices, health history, current health status, and environmental influences as they relate to increasing or reducing disease risk.

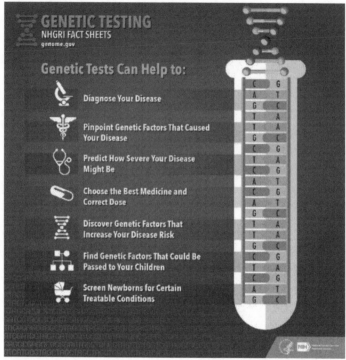

Figure 8: Genetic Testing Example Applications (Source: NHGRI)

Cancer has a major impact on society and expenditures for cancer care in the United States totaled nearly $125 billion in 2010, a figure that could reach $156 billion by 2020. According to the National Cancer Institute, an estimated 1.7 million new cases of cancer were expected to be diagnosed in the United States in 2016, resulting in nearly 600,00 deaths. The most common types of cancer include breast cancer, lung cancer, prostate cancer, colon and rectum cancer, bladder cancer, and melanoma of the skin. Based on 2010-2012 data, nearly 40% of men and women will be diagnosed with cancer at some point during their lifetimes.

For women, a family history of breast and ovarian cancer is important knowledge. Testing of the BRCA1 and BRCA2 gene mutations provides additional, critical insights into the risk for these types of cancer. A recent study confirmed that women with a specific type of the BRCA1 or BRCA2 inherited gene mutation are at increased risk of breast and ovarian cancer and that the magnitude of risk was influenced both by the location of the mutations within the BRCA genes as well as the extent of family history of breast cancer. Moreover, women already diagnosed with cancer can benefit from genetic testing, which can help guide treatment and prevention efforts.

In 2013, Hollywood actress Angelina Jolie publicly revealed her decision to have a double mastectomy based on her BRCA1 positivity and family history of cancer. According to Jolie, "My doctors estimated that I had an 87% risk of breast cancer and a 50% risk of ovarian cancer, although the risk is different in the case of each woman. Once I knew that this was my reality, I decided to be proactive and to minimize the risk as much I could. I made a decision to have a preventive double mastectomy."

Jolie's decision generated considerable media attention for BRCA genetic testing. According to one study, this resulted in a measurable increase in public awareness, with approximately 20% of women indicating that media coverage of Jolie's decision affected their interest in breast cancer.

As it turns out, Jolie's cancer risk may not have been quite as high as originally estimated. Research published in 2017 identified 18 new genetic variations—in addition to BRCA1 and BRCA2—which provide additional information that could help reduce the number of women needing breast-removal surgery by around 33%. Conducted by the Manchester University NHS Foundation Trust (MFT) and the University of Manchester in the UK, the study tested the DNA of 451 women who had developed breast cancer and had a family history of the disease. This information and other factors were used to determine an overall risk estimate for breast cancer. With this new test, women like Jolie might be reclassified to a lower cancer-risk category, reducing the likelihood that they would pursue elective preventive breast-removal surgery.

Genome Sequencing

In the context of disease risk identification and disease prevention, genome sequencing is also beginning to demonstrate medical utility when used for individual patients. Unlike genetic testing—aka genotyping, which determines specific genetic variants possessed by an individual—genome sequencing looks at the order of DNA nucleotides—the four-base code of ACGs and Ts—in an organism's genome.

In 2012, Michael Snyder, PhD, a professor of genetics at Stanford University School of Medicine and director of the Center for Genomics and Personalized

Medicine, reported that, as a result of sequencing his own genome, he had discovered he had a high risk for developing Type 2 diabetes. According to Snyder: "The disease doesn't run in the family and I'm a touch on the thin side, so I don't fit the usual stereotype."

Nonetheless, testing of Snyder's blood over a 14-month period revealed—at a very early stage—that he had developed diabetes. The tests, which looked at ribonucleic acid (RNA, a DNA photocopy of a cell), proteins, metabolites, and autoantibodies, helped catch the disease much earlier than is typical in healthcare today. Snyder used this information to successfully reverse his diabetes through lifestyle behavior change: he eliminated desserts and exercised more. Snyder's study—in which he was both lead author and subject—showed the value of combining genome sequencing and blood tests.

Gene Editing

Because the DNA in our cells contains a digital code, it is now possible to make precise changes to it via a new technology called CRISPR-Cas9 genome editing. CRISPR—which stands for Clustered Regularly Interspaced Short Palindromic Repeats—is a tool that allows geneticists and medical researchers to remove, add, or alter sections in a sequence of DNA. An animated explainer video by Nature can be viewed here.

Recently, researchers from the Lewis Katz School of Medicine at Temple University and the University of Pittsburgh used CRISPR to excise HIV DNA from the genomes of mice, thereby eliminating further infection.

This is significant because the HIV virus can remain dormant in the body for long periods of time and is difficult to eliminate.

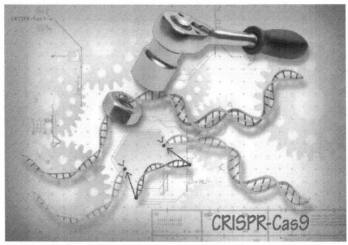

Figure 9: CRISPR-Cas9 (Source: NHGRI)

Another application for CRISPR is germline gene modification, which involves making changes to human embryos or sex cells (sperm and eggs) that can be passed along to the next generation. While this application of CRISPR is currently banned in the United States, a new consensus study by the National Academy of Sciences (NAS) has endorsed it for use in humans, but only in a very narrow application: preventing the birth of children with serious diseases. Harvard Medical School geneticist and genomics pioneer George Church, PhD projects that CRISPR gene-edited sperm could have a role in 6% of births.

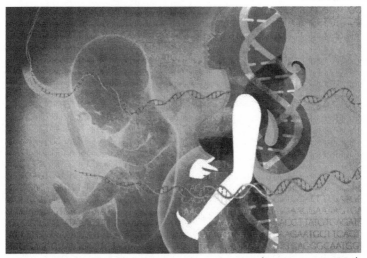

Figure 10: Prenatal Genome Sequencing (Source: NHGRI)

The National Academy of Sciences (NAS) further states that there should be stringent oversight and that enhancements—like attempting to alter genes to make people more intelligent, thereby creating so-called 'designer babies'—should not be pursued at this time. However, biologist Paul Knoepfler, PhD feels that in just over a decade from now we'll start seeing upgrades of this type being made to human embryos. As Knoepfler predicts in his TEDx talk, germline gene modification will be used for everything from altering physical appearance, to increasing intelligence, to eliminating the risk of auto-immune diseases.

The ethical and societal implications of germline gene modification are profound, in large part because the changes are heritable (passable to future generations), thereby altering the evolutionary path of the human species. In 2017, the first known attempt at creating genetically modified human embryos occurred in the United States when a team of researchers at Oregon Health and Science University used CRISPR to change the DNA of a large number of one-cell embryos. The embryos, however, were allowed to develop for only a few days and were never implanted into a womb.

Gene Therapy

Gene therapy is a technique that uses genes—instead of drugs or surgery—to treat or prevent disease. Approaches include replacing a disease-causing mutated gene with a healthy copy of the gene, inactivating (knocking out) an improperly functioning gene, and introducing a new gene into the body to fight a disease. The replacement is accomplished intravenously (IV) or with an injection directly into body tissue, where it is taken up by the cells. Alternatively, a patient's own cells can be removed, exposed to a vector (a virus can be used for this purpose), and then returned to the patient, where the new gene will now make a functioning protein.

While gene therapy holds promise as a treatment option for many diseases—from inherited genetic disorders, to cancer, and even some viral infections—it is currently only being tested for diseases that have no other available cures. In the illustration below, a new gene is shown being injected into an adenovirus vector, which is used to introduce the modified DNA into a human cell. If the treatment is successful, the new gene will make a functional protein.

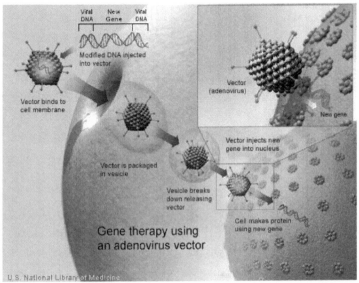

Figure 11: Gene Therapy Using an Adenovirus Vector (Source: U.S. National Library of Medicine)

In 2017, the FDA began approving the first gene therapies. The very first was Novartis' Kymriah, a treatment that genetically modifies a patient's own immune cells (T cells) to fight acute lymphoblastic leukemia, an often-deadly type of blood and bone marrow cancer. The T cells are altered with a new gene that codes for a protein called a chimeric antigen receptor (CAR), giving the treatment its name: CAR-T therapy. The modified protein now directs the T cells to target and kill leukemia cells. The second approval by the FDA was for Gilead Science company Kite Pharma's Yescarta, a cell-based gene therapy to treat adult patients with certain types of non-Hodgkin lymphoma (NHL), a type of immune system cancer.

In a statement regarding the approval of Yescarta, FDA commissioner Dr. Scott Gottlieb said: "We're entering a new frontier in medical innovation with the ability to reprogram a patient's own cells to attack a deadly cancer. Today marks another milestone in the development of a whole new scientific paradigm for the treatment of serious diseases. In just several decades, gene therapy has gone from being a promising concept to a practical solution to deadly and largely untreatable forms of cancer. This approval demonstrates the continued momentum of this promising new area of medicine and we're committed to supporting and helping expedite the development of these products. We will soon release a comprehensive policy to address how we plan to support the development of cell-based regenerative medicine."

While not yet approved at this time, another gene therapy treatment has been unanimously recommended for approval by an FDA advisory panel. Luxturna from Spark Therapeutics is a corrective gene therapy indicated for use in the treatment of certain forms of blindness. While the treatment does not result in 20/20 vision—or work in all cases—it has resulted in improved vision for nearly all the patients treated with it. Luxturna modifies a mutated gene (RPE65) that provides instructions for making a protein necessary for normal vision. Jeff Marrazzo, CEO at Spark Therapeutics, says that the approval of Luxturna would mark a new era in medicine and that: "This is what I believe medicine is going to be like for the next 20, 30, if not 50 years. I think this is the beginning of an age that is going to fundamentally change medicine."

Liquid Biopsies

A liquid biopsy involves the genetic testing or genomic sequencing of a blood sample to look for cancer cells or cancer DNA that is circulating in the blood. The major benefit of a liquid biopsy is that it can identify cancer in its earliest stages, before symptoms appear, and when it is most likely that treatment and other preventive measures will be successful. In some cases, early cancer detection is tantamount to a cure. GRAIL, a genomics company developing these types of tests, even states that its mission is "to detect cancer early, when it can be cured."

In a recent example of the potential for liquid biopsies to save lives and reduce healthcare costs, Dennis Lo, PhD and a team of researchers at Chinese University of Hong Kong screened 20,000 men at risk for nasopharyngeal cancer, a particularly aggressive form of cancer that's common among middle-aged Chinese men. Of those screened, 34 turned out to have the disease, which forms at the top of the throat behind the nose. The study identified the cancer at the earliest stage with a success rate of 71%, versus just 20% for conventional screening methods. When detected early, this cancer can often be cured with radiation alone. But when it is advanced, chemotherapy may be needed, and outcomes are often less successful. Importantly, the screening appeared to improve how many of the men survived without the disease becoming worse, with 97% still being alive after three years compared to 70% among the comparison group.

Imaging

Ultrasound imaging, aka sonography, uses high-frequency sound waves to provide a real-time view inside the body. Movement of the internal organs and blood flow is also visible. One of the added upsides of ultrasound is that, unlike X-ray imaging, there is no ionizing radiation exposure. According to the World Health Organization (WHO), low doses of ionizing radiation—which is also emitted by natural sources including soil, air, food, water, and cosmic rays—can increase the risk of longer term effects such as cancer. The more ionizing radiation one is exposed to, the more potential for health hazards.

As the FDA explains, in a medical ultrasound exam, a transducer probe is placed directly on the skin (or inside a body opening) and a thin layer of gel is applied so that the ultrasound waves are transmitted from the transducer through the gel into the body. The ultrasound image is produced based on the reflection of the waves off structures inside the body. The strength of the sound signal—and the time it takes for the wave to travel through the body—provide the information used to produce an image. Ultrasound imaging can help a physician evaluate, diagnose, and treat a variety medical conditions. These uses and applications include:

- Abdominal ultrasound
- Bone sonometry
- Breast ultrasound

- Doppler ultrasound (to visualize blood flow through a blood vessel, organs, or other structures)
- Echocardiogram (to view the heart)
- Fetal ultrasound (to view the fetus in pregnancy)
- Doppler fetal heart rate monitors
- Ultrasound-guided biopsies (to collect a sample of tissue)
- Ophthalmic ultrasound (to visualize ocular structures)
- Ultrasound-guided needle placement (in blood vessels or other tissues of interest)

In October 2017, Butterfly Network—a company founded by genome sequencing pioneer Jonathan Rothberg, PhD—announced that it had received FDA clearance for its Butterfly iQ ultrasound device that attaches to an iPhone. According to the company, iQ is the world's first ultrasound-on-a-chip based imaging system. Unlike current ultrasound systems—which rely on vibrating piezoelectric crystals to generate sound waves and can cost anywhere from $6,000 for a handheld version to $100,000 for a high-end machine—the iQ, which costs much less, uses nearly 10,000 tiny sensor drums etched onto a semiconductor chip, which send sound waves into the body and capture the returning signals, or echoes.

In describing the unique value provided by the device, the company's Chief Medical Officer, John Martin, MD, stated: "Offering a unique blend of affordability, diagnostic versatility, and assistive intelligence, Butterfly has the potential to impact human health more profoundly than any diagnostic device since the stethoscope, invented over 200 years ago. At less than $2,000, healthcare providers can purchase an easy-to-use, powerful, whole-body medical imaging system that fits in their pocket. By removing the barrier of price, I expect Butterfly to ultimately replace the stethoscope in the daily practice of medicine. We can now provide a diagnostic system to address the millions of children that die of pneumonia each year and the hundreds of thousands of women that die in childbirth, and these are just two examples of the impact this technology will have."

In an interview, Martin says that the device—which he used to diagnose squamous-cell cancer in his own throat—could even be modified into a wearable patch, which patients could wear after leaving the hospital. It might also be used in the home to diagnose bone fractures.

According to market research firm IHS Markit, the global market for ultrasound devices was $5.8 billion in 2013. By moving to all-digital technology, Butterfly Network illustrates another example of digital health disrupting the healthcare status quo by lowering costs, improving portability, increasing access, and delivering higher quality care. Rothberg emphasizes these points, saying: "Just as putting a camera on a semiconductor chip made photography accessible to anyone with a smart phone and putting a computer on a chip enabled the revolution in personal computing before that, Butterfly's ultrasound-on-a-chip technology enables a low-cost window into the human body, making high-quality diagnostic imaging accessible to anyone. Two thirds of the world's population has no access to medical imaging, that's not ok, and today our team is doing something about it. And they are just getting started."

Autonomous Vehicles

Air pollution kills about 7 million people worldwide each year, with more than half of the fatalities due to fumes from indoor stoves, according to a report from the World Health Organization (WHO). Self-driving cars can reduce the pollution caused by automobiles in addition to providing other health and lifesaving benefits.

It's estimated that self-driving cars, aka autonomous vehicles, could save 300,000 lives per decade in the United States by decreasing traffic fatalities. This is comparable to the life-saving benefits of modern vaccines, which save about 42,000 lives each year in the U.S. With about 1.2 million traffic fatalities each year around the world, extrapolating the U.S. benefits equates to driverless cars saving 10 million lives per decade, globally. Moreover, the potential exists for reducing U.S. roadway crashes by 90%, which would result in a savings of around $190 billion per year in associated healthcare costs.

Autonomous vehicles could also reduce CO_2 greenhouse gas emissions by 90% while consuming nearly 100% less oil than gas-powered vehicles. It's estimated that driverless cars will represent 10% of global vehicle sales, or about 12 million cars sold per year by 2035.

Transportation infrastructure and vehicles are also beginning to communicate with one another, providing benefits in addition to those mentioned above. The U.S. Department of Transportation (DOT) has proposed new Vehicle to Vehicle (V2V) rules, which would have cars share data with each other via short-range communication channels. Broadcasted data would include location, direction, and speed, which would enable cars to warn drivers about dangers they were unable to see or perceive. V2V sensors would also provide information to autonomous vehicles for use in helping them brake, slow, or turn to prevent a collision. We can expect a future of chatty cars that—unlike humans— are safer as a result. The DOT says that V2V could prevent hundreds of thousands of crashes every year.

An added complementary layer of information is also arriving from the Federal Highway Administration, which plans to issue guidance for Vehicle-to-Infrastructure (V2I) communications. V2I allows vehicles to communicate with roadway infrastructure such as traffic lights, stop signs, and work zones, which would improve mobility, reduce congestion, and improve safety.

Human Augmentation

Human augmentation—via digital technologies and genomics—offers incredible potential to enhance our mental and physical capabilities, possibly even extend our lives. Applications fall across a wide spectrum and include uses for the able-bodied and people with disabilities.

Implantable radio-frequency identification (RFID) computer chips, while approved by the FDA for over 15 years, have once again been making headlines. In 2004, the Verichip, made by Applied Digital Systems, was approved for use in patients so that their medical records and other vital medical information could be rapidly accessed if a patient is unconscious, uncommunicative, or lacks medical records. The company had already been given the green light a couple of years before by the FDA for non-medical applications of its device.

Another company, Three Square Market, recently claimed to be the first U.S. company to provide RFID implants to its employees. CEO Todd Westby believes that this technology will soon be commonplace, saying: "We foresee the use of RFID technology to drive everything from making purchases in our office break room market, opening doors, use of copy machines, logging into our office computers, unlocking phones, sharing business cards, storing medical/health information, and used as payment at other RFID terminals. Eventually, this technology will become standardized, allowing you to use this as your passport, public transit, all purchasing opportunities, etc." Considering the safety and privacy concerns expressed by some, Westby adds that "The chip is not trackable and only contains information you choose to associate with it. This chip does not have GPS capabilities."

Robotic exoskeletons, which enhance physical body strength, offer a wide variety of applications: from assisting the elderly; people with injuries, disabilities, or muscle weakness; and helping workers to perform better and reduce their risk of injury. Ekso Bionics, which originally developed their exoskeleton suits to help soldiers carry heavy loads, has repurposed their products to help victims of stroke, traumatic brain injury (TBI), and people who have suffered spinal cord injuries. According to CEO Nathan Harding, rehabilitation clinics are using the company's exoskeletons to help get patients moving around as soon as possible after an injury, which can improve recovery time. "What's really exciting about our device," he says, "is (patients) can get up and they get usually two or three hundred steps in the very first session."

Another important area of human augmentation involves the use of brain-computer interface (BCI) devices. By providing a direct communication pathway between the brain and external devices, BCIs have applications in research, brain mapping, and assisting human cognitive and sensory-motor functions. For example, a paralyzed man recently became the first person to test a sensory-enhanced robotic hand that also imparted a sense of feel when the hand was being touched. These systems offer a means of restoring the ability to perform independent activities associated with normal daily living to paralyzed people. Simply being able to hold a coffee cup, handle a credit card, or sign a document provides an important sense of independence and self-determination for paralyzed individuals.

Companies like Facebook are also researching the potential for BCIs to enable communications via thought. The noninvasive system they are reportedly exploring might work by using a diffuse optical imaging (DOI) system (sometimes called diffuse optical tomography), which is based on shining near-infrared light onto brain tissue. The way in which the light scatters off brain neurons is measured and associated with a person thinking a word or words previously learned by the system. In addition to the enablement this would provide for people with disabilities, it would also serve as an alternative to voice recognition technologies, which are not always practical or secure when used within earshot of others. Moreover, it would be up to three times faster than typing on a smartphone.

Other companies working on the development of BCIs include Neuralink, founded by Elon Musk (Tesla and SpaceX); Kernel, founded by Bryan Johnson (OS Fund and Braintree); and Openwater, founded by Mary Louise Jepsen (X, Facebook, and Oculus). Details on each of these companies are sparse, but the investments being made are significant and imply enormous opportunities for human augmentation, including—as Kernel is focused on—the reduction of cognitive deficiencies for people with Alzheimer's and dementia. According to Kernel CEO Bryan Johnson, while "individuals facing cognitive deficiencies will be the first super-humans", his intent is "to build products for billions of people, not just elite or rich." He describes additional applications, including the potential to purchase intelligence as well as enable the right of individuals to "self-address diseases like anxiety and depression".

Self-administered gene therapy as a means of human augmentation—as opposed to treating an illness—is in its early, and unregulated days, at least in the United States. One of the pioneers in this area is microbiologist Brian Hanley, PhD, who is injecting gene therapies into his own body in an effort to increase his strength, stamina, and life span. The procedure he uses involves injecting circular DNA plasmid rings of the gene for growth-hormone-releasing hormone (GHRH) into his thigh and then applying an electrical current through electrodes that are stuck into his thighs. The current temporarily opens the cells, permitting the DNA rings to enter them. The cells—which now contain the new DNA in their nuclei—are now programmed to manufacture proteins based on the new code. The effect lasts only a few weeks and the DNA does not become a permanent part of Hanley's chromosomes.

Hanley has been evaluated at George Church's Harvard genomics lab, where elevated levels of GHRH appeared to be present. The Church lab is testing many types of gene therapy in mice to see if their lives can be extended and or even experience a reversal of the aging process. This recalls the movie 'The Curious Case of Benjamin Button', which was about a man—played by Brad Pitt—who starts aging backwards.

Another gene therapy pioneer is Josiah Zayner, PhD, who is using the CRISPR gene editing tool to essentially snip DNA at a specific location and knock out a gene responsible for producing a muscle growth-limiting hormone. In China, a study using this method conducted on dogs resulted in a doubling of their muscle mass.

According to Church, gene therapy is underrated as a means of conquering old age and he predicts that one day everyone will take it, stating: "A scenario is, everyone takes gene therapy—not just curing rare diseases like cystic fibrosis, but diseases that everyone has, like aging. One of our biggest economic disasters right now is our aging population. If we eliminate retirement, then it buys us a couple of decades to straighten out the economies of the world".

Pandemics and Health Testing

The Influenza Pandemic of 1918-1919 infected 500 million people—or 33% of the world's population—and killed approximately 50 million people. It was one of the most devastating pandemics (the worldwide spread of a new disease) in recorded history, killing nearly as many people in a single year as were killed during the 'Black Death' bubonic plague, which occurred in Europe from 1346 to 1353.

In 2009, the H1N1 influenza 'swine flu' virus was detected in the United States and then spread rapidly around the globe, resulting in an estimated 151,700 to 575,400 deaths. The World Health Organization declared it a pandemic virus in the same year. And while hundreds of thousands of people die every year from seasonal flu epidemics, the spread of the virus is limited because many people already have some immunity to it and seasonal influenza vaccines are produced to help reduce illness and deaths.

The reason for the quick spread and devastating impact of the pandemic H1N1 virus was that it was a new virus—a unique combination of influenza genes never previously identified in either animals or people—and most people had little or no immunity to it.

Moreover, there was no vaccine at the outset of the pandemic, as the 2009 H1N1 virus was <u>not</u> included in the manufacturing of 2009-2010 seasonal flu vaccine because it wasn't identified until after manufacturers had started production. <u>Manufacturing</u> of flu pandemic vaccine typically takes several months from the time the virus is identified. In the case of H1N1, the vaccine did not become available until two months <u>after</u> the pandemic had peaked.

Fortunately, this situation is likely to change in the near future. J. Craig Venter is spearheading a new, digital process that can cut the time to produce a new vaccine down to just a few <u>days</u>. The Biomedical Advanced Research and Development Authority (BARDA), the Novartis Foundation, and the National Institute of Allergy and Infectious Diseases (NIAID) are funding work being done by the Venter Institute, Synthetic Genomics, and Novartis that involves digitizing viral genomes to reproduce—or 'rescue'—flu viruses in just over four days.

According to Venter, the digitized virus genome information is sent via the Internet to a Novartis manufacturing facility, where the vaccine is rapidly synthesized and immediately goes into production. Venter indicates that: "If it's a really egregious pandemic, I think we can get it down to six weeks." This compares very favorably to the approximately nine months it took to develop, manufacture, and distribute the H1N1 vaccine.

An essential device enabling this new process is Venter's Digital-to-Biological Converter (DBC), a device that reconstructs binary digital representations of DNA's chemical building blocks, those four base pairs of digital code: adenine (A), cytosine (C), guanine (G), and thymine (T). As Venter explains it, the DBC is just like a printer—in that it uses cassettes—but instead of colors, the cartridges hold bottles of chemicals to print DNA, RNA (key for decoding DNA instructions), viruses, some vaccines, and bacteriophages to kill infections. It can also print simple synthetic bacterium. The hope is that the DBC will one day be deployed in hospitals, clinics, businesses, and even homes, so that if a viral outbreak hits, the specific vaccine can be rapidly developed and then sent digitally anywhere on the planet to stop pandemics in their tracks.

SpaceX's Elon Musk has reportedly expressed interest in using a DBC to print bacteria for use in terraforming Mars. And Martian colonists would likely need vaccines, antibiotics, and personalized drugs, which could also be sent to them digitally. In the event that DNA-based life is discovered on Mars, it could be digitized and transmitted back to Earth, where scientists could recreate the organisms here on Earth. Feel free to insert your own science fiction horror movie script, here!

In the less-distant future, the DBA may soon be used in medical care here on Earth. For example, it could be used to print out the DNA that encodes the hormone insulin, which can be added to a protein synthesis kit used to create insulin for injection. There's also an opportunity to address the antibiotic resistance crisis by using naturally occurring viruses—known as bacteriophages or phages—that kill specific bacteria. Prior to the advent of penicillin, this was actually a common practice used in Russia and Eastern Europe for treating infections. According to Venter, the DBC can be used to sequence the genome of a bacterial infection in just a few minutes and, armed with this genomic information, a phage can be designed to attack specific bacteria that has infected someone.

Virus detection devices—serving as precursors to the DBC—are also set to arrive in our homes. While comparatively limited in functionality, these health-testing and medical diagnostic tools are establishing a new digital health market category and paving the way for future systems like the DBC. Our homes could become self-contained systems providing diagnostic testing and medical treatment. This represents a disintermediation of lab testing, healthcare facilities (hospitals and doctors' offices), and pharmaceutical drug-makers.

A company named Cue, which received media coverage in 2014—but appears to have since gone dark in terms of publicity—is developing a cartridge-based biosensor and microfluidics system for testing blood, saliva, and nasal swab biological samples for use in 'deep health tracking'. Information imparted to consumers includes body inflammation (an indication of recovery from workouts), vitamin D levels, fertility (indicated by the luteinizing hormone), influenza, and testosterone, as can be seen in this promotional video. A companion smartphone app would guide users to optimize their lifestyle behaviors based on this data.

According to an update on the company's website, it is now focused on developing its technology beyond what it initially set out to do regarding infectious disease testing. The statement reads: "Cue can now detect the actual DNA or RNA of an infectious agent. We developed our own nucleic acid amplification technology to help enhance sensitivity for tests such as influenza, HIV, strep throat, chlamydia, (and) gonorrhea. As part of this capability, we began a partnership with Johnson & Johnson to develop a quantitative HIV viral load test especially focused on the developing world."

Coincidentally, Cue was formed in 2009 during the period of the H1N1 flu pandemic. Cue also happens to be based in San Diego, CA, where much of Venter's DBC work is taking place.

Another example of an at-home health-monitoring solution that may arrive on the market soon is called Cor. The company was founded by Bob Messerschmidt who, after selling his previous company to Apple, led the development of the heart rate sensor in the first-generation Apple Watch. The Cor device uses vibrational spectroscopic technology to test a tiny sample of your blood for cholesterol (HDL, LDL, and total), fasting blood glucose, inflammation (fibrinogen protein), and triglycerides. These health indicators are used to provide personalized recommendations on diet, supplements, exercise, and relaxation, with the objective of helping users reach or maintain their health and wellness goals. Fibrinogen is a key regulator of inflammation in disease and can be useful informative for people who perform intense fitness training.

Cor's website points out that while many of us track steps, exercise, sleep, weight, and diet, it asks: "Do you know if these things are making you healthier?" Cor adds that, with their system: "You can finally see which efforts make a real difference in your health."

A few other at-home and mail-in lab testing service providers include:

- myLAB Box – Provides screening solutions for sexually transmitted diseases and infections (STDs & STIs), including HIV (I & II), Hepatitis C, Herpes type-II, Syphilis, Chlamydia, Gonorrhea, Trichomoniasis, Mycoplasma genitalium, and HPV. Sample collection kits are ordered online and mailed back to the company for testing, which also provides free telehealth physician consultations. According to the CDC, STDs—such as chlamydia, gonorrhea, syphilis, and trichomoniasis—can all be treated and cured with antibiotics, which are safe to take during pregnancy. Viral STDs, however—including genital herpes, hepatitis B, and HIV—cannot be cured.

- EverlyWell – Offers a wide variety of tests that consumers can order via its website, including food sensitivity, thyroid, metabolism, men's health, women's health and fertility, sexually transmitted diseases and infections (STDs & STIs), and heavy metals.

- WellnessFX – Analyzes a wide variety of blood biomarkers, including those related to energy and metabolism, strength and endurance, bone and muscle health, brain and body, oxygen and performance, inflammation, minerals, liver health, and blood count. Tests are ordered online, but blood is drawn at a laboratory facility or in your home by a licensed phlebotomist.

- InsideTracker – Analyzes a wide variety of blood biomarkers, including those related to liver and kidney health, performance hormones (which effect muscle growth, fat storage, mood, and libido), metabolic hormones, thyroid function and blood sugar, blood count and nutrients, and cholesterol. The company also offers a women's reproductive panel and consultations with physicians. Tests are ordered online, but blood is drawn at a laboratory facility.

- YO – Enables men to perform a sperm 'selfie' at home using the YO device and a smartphone. Information imparted includes sperm volume and motility, which are key indicators of sperm health.

- Future Family – Provides insights to women into how their fertility is tracking relative to their age and the status of ovarian reserve (how many eggs they have left).

- Teloyears – The company analyzes your DNA and measures the length of your telomeres from a blood sample you mail in. According to the company and emerging research, telomeres are the protective caps on your DNA strands that grow or shrink as a result of good or bad lifestyle factors like chronic stress, sleep quality, exercise, nutrition, chemical intake, and even strained relationships. The company offers a personalized set of suggestions to improve your lifestyle, vitality, and telomere health.

Food Security

According to the Food and Agriculture Organization of the United Nations (FAO), while there is more than enough food produced in the world to feed everyone, over 800 million people still go hungry. And after a decade of decline, global hunger is once again on the rise, affecting 11% of the global population. With global population expected to increase from 7.6 billion people currently to around 10 billion by 2050, one of the greatest challenges we face is producing enough food to meet the nutritional needs for an additional 2.4 billion people. To do so, global food production will have to increase by 50% globally.

The FAO adds that food security is a complex condition requiring a holistic approach to all forms of malnutrition, including the productivity and incomes of small-scale food producers, increased resilience of food production systems (for example due to climate change and competition for resources like water), and the sustainable use of biodiversity and genetic resources.

The latter point about genetic resources is apropos of the genomic aspects of digital health, which offer the potential to create a second agricultural revolution. The gene editing tool CRISPR has applications in food production and improving farm animal production and welfare. As Mick Watson, PhD, a professor of genomics and bioinformatics at The Roslin Institute within The University of Edinburgh points out, since the 1960s, selective breeding (not genetic modification) has significantly increased the production of the food system. For example, in pigs, the percentage of lean meat produced per ton of feed has increased 100% during the past 45 years. But, he says, we still need to keep going to meet growing food demands.

In another presentation, Watson points out that there are opportunities to decrease methane gas produced by cows and other ruminants—animals like cows, sheep, goats, deer—which have complex digestive systems containing a ruminal microbiome optimized to extract energy and nutrition from plant materials. Watson states that there are 270 million dairy cows in the world producing 770 billion liters of milk per year, which is valued at $328B. There are around 570 million farms in the world, with 1-in-4 involved in milk production. Most of these farms have just one or two milk and dairy animals, which provide a key route out of poverty for low- and middle-income countries. Ruminants are the major producers of methane, a greenhouse gas that traps heat in the atmosphere and contributes to global warming at a rate that is 25 times higher than that of carbon dioxide (CO_2). Watson's work at The Roslin Institute involves both trying to increase farm animal food production (like milk) with the same amount of food input plus attempting to find novel enzymes in the ruminant microbiome for use in biofuels production and reduction of methane emissions.

Monsanto—a producer of genetically engineered (GE) seed and herbicides—has entered into an agreement with the Broad Institute of MIT and Harvard to license the new CRISPR-Cpf1 genome editing technology in agriculture. The new system has potential to be a simpler and more precise tool for making targeted improvements in a cell's DNA when compared to the CRISPR-Cas9 system. Tom Adams, PhD, biotechnology lead for Monsanto, stated that "This system offers a technical step-change by presenting new ways to improve crops for farmers and society alike, offering researchers greater flexibility and new capabilities using this emerging technology to improve agriculture." Monsanto has also licensed CRISPR-Cas9 from the Broad Institute.

DuPont Pioneer—also a producer of genetically modified organisms (GMOs), including crops with insect and herbicide resistance—recently secured exclusive rights to CRISPR gene-editing technology for agricultural uses and applications in plants. While company VP Neal Gutterson says, "We see CRISPR-Cas technology as an advancement in plant breeding which can enable a new era in crop improvement", Antonio Regalado, senior editor for biomedicine at MIT Technology Review, pointed out on Twitter that the "First DuPont CRISPR product is a waxier corn, useful as emulsifier for salad dressing. Not quite stopping world hunger yet either." The critique on the yet-to-be-realized potential of gene editing to significantly increase agricultural production is worth noting.

Curious about the apparent duplication of CRISPR patents and licensing by DuPont Pioneer and Monsanto, I asked Regalado if these are different. He responded that they are: "Competing sets of IP (intellectual property) covering (the) same tech." While there had been a major legal challenge over the ownership of CRISPR patents resulting from invention of the technology, the U.S. Patent Office ruled in favor of the Broad Institute, allowing it to retain the patents covering the use of CRISPR in human and animal cells. However, the University of California, Berkeley has filed an appeal.

Some noteworthy genetically modified foods include golden rice, which has been engineered to contain beta-carotene, a precursor of vitamin A. An estimated 670,000 children under the age of 5 die each year because of this dietary deficiency. Rice is the staple food for more than half of the world's population and makes up approximately 50% of the daily energy intake for millions of people living in poverty in Asian countries. It is also becoming an important food staple in Latin America and Africa.

And a Golden Delicious variety of apple that's been genetically engineered to never brown will hit the shelves of U.S. supermarkets beginning in November of 2017. According to Neal Carter, president of Okanagan Specialty Fruits, the Arctic Apple was conceived as a way of increasing apple consumption and decreasing apple waste: "There's an awful lot of apples that go to waste," Carter told Gizmodo from the midst of the apple harvest at his company farm in British Columbia. "We've seen apple consumption decline on a per capita basis over the last few decades, because they're not seen as convenient. When they started selling cut baby carrots, it more than doubled consumption. We were looking for ways to rebrand apples to make them more convenient." Unlike many previous forms of genetically engineered foods like corn, the Arctic is not transgenic, meaning it does not contain a gene from another species. This type of gene alteration may prove to be more palatable to consumers than a tomato with flounder genes. A bruise-resistant Innate potato that's also non-transgenic is already on shelves.

J. Craig Venter has even stated that he is trying to make meat by making beef and chicken muscle proteins without using actual cows and chickens. He calls it "motherless meat" and then Brian Eno calls it "murderless" meat. According to Venter, "Those of you who are vegetarians are going to have real dilemmas in the future of not knowing what's meat and what's vegetable, because in fact, we can grow these meat proteins in vegetables. In fact, vegetables have most of the same proteins that are in meat anyway. Our definitions of life are getting clearer; the social ambiguities are getting greater."

In July of 2017, the U.S. Department of Agriculture approved a proposal by Cornell University to use genetically engineered, self-destructing moths in upstate New York as a pesticide-free way of fighting crop damage caused by the diamondback moth. This invasive species eats cabbage, cauliflower, and broccoli. According to Emily Mullin, at MIT Technology Review, this would be "the first open-air release of genetically modified insects created with a technology other than radiation for agriculture in the U.S."

Satellites, robots, and drones are also changing the future of agriculture. The University of Sydney's Australian Centre for Field Robotics is developing methods for robotic farming that include driverless tractors, which can drive over crops, gather data for farmers, and even perform tasks like spraying, weeding, trimming branches, and harvesting fruits. Drones can perform similar and additional tasks, including planting, soil health scans, pest and disease detection, monitoring crop health, applying fertilizers, watering fields, weather tracking, and yield estimates. Satellites are also being used for soil and analysis of crop and production inefficiencies, for use in improving crop management.

Artificial intelligence (AI) is also being applied to advance agriculture. A new partnership between Monsanto and Atomwise seeks to speed the discovery of molecules that help protect crops. It's hoped that deep learning algorithms will cut the development time and cost for bringing new pest- and disease-resistant crops to market.

There are many more opportunities to increase food production, produce crops with greater and added nutrients, require less nitrogen fertilizers, improve drought and moisture resilience, decrease food waste, and increase resistance to diseases and pests, all of which bear promise for addressing the growing challenges of food security in the face of an expanding global population and the impact of climate change on agriculture.

The Fourth Wave

Over the past 12,000 years, there have been three great waves of human progress linked to major technological innovations: The Agricultural Revolution, the Industrial Age, and the Digital Revolution.

Waves of Human and Technological Progress

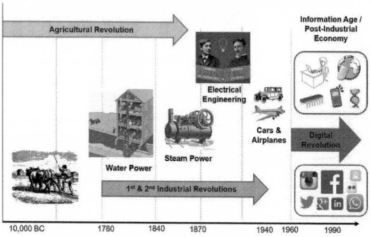

Figure 12: Waves of Human and Technological Progress (Source: Paul Sonnier)

One way of describing these waves of human progress—or sociocultural evolution—is a term coined by economist Joseph Schumpeter, who called it "creative destruction", a process by which the entire modus operandi of society—from the economy, to culture, and even political mechanisms—are fundamentally transformed. (Topol pays homage to

Schumpeter in his book, 'The Creative Destruction of Medicine'.)

Another perspective was popularized by futurist Alvin Toffler, whose 1980 bestseller, 'The Third Wave', described the Digital Revolution as bringing about the Third Wave of society. (Steve Case pays homage to Toffler in his book of the same name.) According to Toffler: "You don't just make technological changes without also making social changes. (You) cannot have a new economy without also getting a new society."

Toffler describes the First Wave as the society that came into being during The Agricultural Revolution, aka the Neolithic Revolution, which was the period starting around 12,000 years ago when agrarian society began replacing hunter-gatherer cultures.

The Second Wave is the society that developed during the Industrial Age, beginning around 1760, with the transition from hand production methods to machines, the use of water and steam power, the emergence of the factory system, and development of new manufacturing and production processes. Later, in the second phase of the Industrial Revolution— beginning about 1850—electricity and petroleum became important sources of energy (for lighting, small motors, autos, and trucks), with advances in communications, electrical engineering, science, and medicine all combining to create widespread changes in society.

The Third Wave society was initiated by the Digital Revolution—aka Information Age or Post-Industrial Economy/Society—beginning around the late 1950s and is the result of the invention and large-scale adoption of digital logic circuits and derivative technologies such as the computer, digital cellular phone, and the Internet.

In his book, Toffler also includes genomics within the bounds of the Information Age, saying that: "Just as the Second Wave combined coal, steel, electricity, and rail transport to produce automobiles and a thousand other life-transforming products, the real impact of the new changes will not be felt until we reach the stage of combining the new technologies—linking together computers, electronics, new materials from outer space and the oceans, with genetics, and all of these, in turn, with the new energy base. Bringing these elements together will release a flood of innovation unlike any seen before in human history. We are constructing a dramatically new techno-sphere for a Third Wave civilization."

However, in a 1997 WIRED piece, Toffler—who, unfortunately, never wrote 'The Fourth Wave'—was quoted as saying: "Those of us who are monitoring social change and the meaning of being human have a major agenda item planted right smack in front of us. We have barely begun to absorb the impact of the Third Wave—and we're now facing the next, (the Fourth Wave, which) combines information technology with the genetic advances that we've made into a completely new wave of social, political, religious, ethical, and legal changes."

It is this latter statement—made by Toffler 17 years after publication of 'The Third Wave'—that eloquently describes the new era of human progress we are entering: The Fourth Wave. Software, digital devices, sensors, and sensing systems (which includes data and software-derived information gathering systems) are becoming ever more integral and pervasive in our lives. Moreover, these tools can work passively and unobtrusively, which increases their utility in an increasing number of applications.

Genetic testing and sequencing, as well, continue to provide increasing value as costs drop. This forms a virtuous cycle, wherein more people are tested and sequenced, which generates additional valuable information, in turn providing more incentives for stakeholders to do more testing. Like the emergence of the app economy, there is now an emerging opportunity for genomic app stores. One such entity providing this platform is Illumina-spinout company Helix, which offers a one-stop shop for leveraging both our own and the vast and growing pools of genomic insights and complementary services being offered by third parties.

Digital tools for our health and healthcare are already in, on, and connected to our smartphones. They are now beginning to enter our homes as standalone devices, which feature monitoring and testing of our health, medical diagnostics, including genetic testing.

Public health surveillance via digital disease detection—which uses explicit or inferential data about diseases and outbreaks disseminated by governments and NGOs, plus in press reports, blogs, chat rooms, Web searches, and social media—can reduce the time to recognize disease outbreaks. Moreover, technology like that found in Oxford Nanopore's MinION promises to one day deliver genomic sequencing and testing embedded in devices that we use every day. This would provide <u>genomics-informed</u>, real-time public health surveillance of pathogens (bacteria, viruses, or other microorganisms that can cause disease) with the potential for viral genome sequence data, for example, to be sent to Venter's Digital-to-Biological Converter (DBC) located in your home. At that stage, a vaccine could be tailored to your genome and environment, printed, and consumed, thereby stopping a pandemic in its tracks.

As Toffler points out, the combination of digital technology and genomics will create—in addition to health and medical system changes—a completely new wave of social, political, religious, ethical, and legal changes.

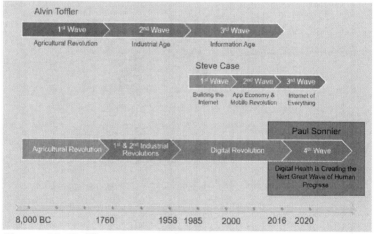

Figure 13: Toffler, Case, and Sonnier Waves (Source: Paul Sonnier)

Timeline

When will the Fourth Wave happen? Previous great changes wrought upon society by technological innovation and adoption have taken as long as thousands of years to manifest (the Agricultural Revolution), to hundreds (the Industrial Era), and now decades (the Digital Revolution). Changes can be very diffuse, with some populations, industry sectors, geographic regions of the globe, and healthcare systems, to name a few, advancing at different speeds. As science fiction writer William Gibson famously stated, "The future is already here—it's just not very evenly distributed."

As I've highlighted via examples—and in outlining the broad categories and impact areas of digital health—the digital and genomic innovations bringing the Fourth Wave into being are already widely used and having measurable impacts throughout society. Even so, as is usually the case with emerging technologies and derived innovations, the distribution of adoption and commensurate benefits are often fragmented. And depending on the type of application and technology, adoption exists at varying degrees of scale: from one person (e.g. what Michael Snyder is doing in his single-person studies) to billions of people (the positives and negatives related to smartphone and mobile app usage).

A good analysis of the rate of adoption and benefits for some key areas of digital health—including underlying and related technologies—comes from consulting firm Gartner. Each year, the company puts out its <u>Hype Cycle for Emerging Technologies</u>, which provides a graphic representation of the maturity and adoption over time of technologies and applications as well as how they are potentially relevant to solving real business problems and exploiting new opportunities. The 'Plateau of Productivity' is how Gartner describes the benchmark for the point at which mainstream adoption starts to take off and the "technology's broad market applicability and relevance are clearly paying off."

In the company's 2017 Hype Cycle, three emerging technology megatrends are highlighted: artificial intelligence (AI), transparently immersive experiences, and digital platforms. Near term, the subcategories of these that are most relevant to digital health fall within these three categories as follows, with their 'Plateau of Productivity' indicated in parentheses:

- Artificial Intelligence (AI)
    - Artificial General Intelligence – more than 10 years
    - Autonomous Vehicles – more than 10 years
    - Smart Robots – 5-10 years
    - Deep & Machine Learning – 2-5 years
    - Cognitive Expert Advisers – 2-5 years
    - Conversational User Interfaces – 5-10 years
    - Virtual Assistants – 5-10 years
    - Drones – 2-5 years
- Transparently Immersive Experiences
    - Augmented Reality (AR) – 5-10 years

- o Brain-Computer Interfaces (BCI) – more than 10 years
- o Human Augmentation – more than 10 years
- o Virtual Reality (VR) – 2-5 years
- o Connected Home – 5-10 years
- Digital Platforms
  - o 5G (5th generation mobile networks) – 5-10 years
  - o Blockchain (to address healthcare data interoperability and data security) – 5-10 years
  - o Internet of Things (IoT) – 2-5 years
  - o Neuromorphic Hardware (computers that imitate the human brain) – 5-10 years

Two noteworthy areas in the above that I have not elaborated on are 5G and virtual reality (VR). These offer important benefits and growing applications for society and across the spectrum of business sectors. Below is an overview of their potential in these areas along with market size estimates.

5G

5th generation mobile networks will provide vastly greater coverage areas and higher bandwidth, speed, and density of mobile data connections than exist with today's 4G networks. A white paper by the Next Generation Mobile Networks Alliance (NGMN), indicates that 5G will enable a massive growth in the ability for simultaneous connections for users, wireless sensors, cameras, and IoT devices. The mobile and connected society will need broadband access to be available everywhere, and we'll see data rates of balloon to 100 megabits per second. Moreover, deployment of 5G is expected be low cost, thereby offering Internet access in underserved areas of the world. The benefits of this include new business opportunities as well as greater access to healthcare services.

According to a report by market research firm IHA Markit, the 5G value chain will play a central role in enabling $12.3 trillion in global economic output by 2035. In a related report based on IHA Markit's findings, David Teece, PhD, a professor at U.C. Berkeley's Haas School of Business, estimates that the impact of 5G on the healthcare market will amount to more than $1.1 trillion over this same period of time. According to a statement from Qualcomm, 5G will be a "substantial enabler of a new era of "personalized health care" providing the ability to leverage large amounts of patient-specific data to develop predictive analytics and take courses of action tailored to the patient and his or her condition, also giving patients greater ability to manage conditions on their own." Professor Teece adds that "Few people are cognizant of the full impact that the (sic) mobile communications has on their lives or on the economy. There is growing evidence that wireless technology is the silent enabler of technological progress throughout the economy. Health care is a large and growing sector of our economy. Technologies that improve productivity and patient care are much sought after. 5G will open the door to important developments in personalized, anywhere, anytime, medicine."

Virtual Reality

VR offers a wide variety of applications in health and healthcare. In the area of mental health, VR has proven useful in the treatment of Post-Traumatic Stress Disorder (PTSD), phobias, and traumas from sexual assault. It's also been found to help with pain. For example, a trial demonstrated that burn victims immersed in virtual environments experienced 50% less pain during wound care treatment than patients attempting other means of distraction from pain. VR is also being used for health and medical education, including training surgeons and medical students, general training in cardiopulmonary resuscitation (CPR) lifesaving technique, and educating women about child birthing. It is also being investigated for use in diagnosing dementia.

ABI Research projects that VR services in the medical and healthcare segment will grow in value from $8.9 million in 2017 to around $285 million in 2022. Although digital health VR is still a niche segment (overall VR market size is projected to be $34 billion by 2022), ABI sees growing interest and investment in VR applications from professionals, hospitals, and medical institutions driving a significant new wave of applications being used to treat patients around the world.

Genomics

While genomics is not tracked by Gartner as an 'emerging technology', as I've illustrated, genome sequencing and genetic testing continues to expand in terms of consumer, healthcare, and other applications and value provided. The knowledge gained from whole genome sequencing (WGS) is critical input to genetic testing, as the ability to gain new insights—for example, through genome-wide association studies (GWAS) that compare large numbers human genomes—increases in relation to the numbers of people who have had their genome sequenced. In other words, the more genomes used for comparison, the more likely it is that new insights can be found.

GWAS help scientists to gain insights into disease, response to certain drugs, and the interactions between genes and the environment. By searching the genome for small variations called single nucleotide polymorphisms (SNPs)—which occur more frequently in people with a particular disease than in people who don't have the disease—it is possible to pinpoint genes that may contribute to a person's risk of developing certain diseases, including diabetes, heart abnormalities, Parkinson disease, and Crohn disease.

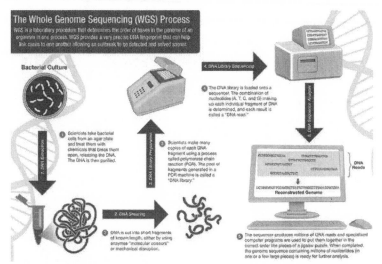

*Figure 14: Whole Genome Sequencing Process Workflow
(Source: CDC)*

A recent article by Preetika Rana in the Wall Street Journal indicates that China and the United States are collecting genetic data from at least 1 million people in each country as part of their respective national precision medicine programs. China is expected to complete their initial collection by 2020, followed by the U.S. in 2022. An important distinction is also noted: Only the U.S. will store the genetic data on a common server, grant participants access to their data analysis, and monitor the lifestyles of patients.

In a January 2017 article by Matthew Herper at Forbes, he reports that, according to Illumina, more than 500,000 human genomes had been sequenced as of that time. It's unclear if this was a total global estimate or only genomes sequenced on Illumina's machines. A

<u>tweet</u> by me at the time—in which I mentioned Illumina, its CEO, Francis deSouza, Matthew Herper, Antonio Regalado, and Mick Watson—only elicited one reply, which was from Regalado, who stated: "let's see how that estimate was reached". So, it seems that the exact number of human genomes sequenced to date is, unfortunately, a bit of a mystery. Even so, it's likely that the number is in the hundreds of thousands. With the public and private sequencing efforts currently underway around the world, the tally will likely reach a million or more by 2020.

Inflection Point

The Digital and Genomic Revolutions are already transforming all sectors of the economy and global society. Taking into consideration Gartner's estimates for relevant emerging technologies to reach their plateaus of productivity—and a similar timeframe for genomics to ramp up in terms of impact—I project that the Fourth Wave will rapidly accelerate beginning in 2020. The critical mass is in place and it seems likely that at that point in time, the convergence of many key factors will create a perfect storm catalyzing digital health.

Businesses and Organizations

From a business and organizational perspective, strategies for success in digital health—while not cookie-cooker—fall within the four general types: Enhancement, Multifaceted, Adjacent, and Disruption.

It's important to reiterate that these approaches—as well as the varied efforts being pursued by healthcare providers—are all valid and worthy of being pursued. Moreover, even for business entities, success does not always entail a direct focus on revenue and profit. Leveraging digital health to improve people's lives, enhance society, and improve healthcare can be a strategic addition to a portfolio that helps grow other lines of business. It can also provide humanitarian benefits as a corporate social responsibility (CSR) function.

When considering a digital health strategy, it helps to keep in mind a few key focus areas for businesses and organizations. Again, these are not a fit for all entities and there are often overlaps:

- The provision of disease diagnosis, management, prediction, and prevention (whether explicit or not)
- Large scale digital customer interface
- High intent users
- Agile (critical, but difficult for incumbents)
- Innovation and M&A
- Diversification & new business models
- Ecosystem partnering (innovators and incumbents)
- Platforms (inclusive of ecosystem partners)
- Dislocation of incumbents (disruption)
- Evolution of established players

It's important to point out that no single company or entity is transforming our world and creating the Fourth Wave on their own. Alas, there is no 'Uber of Digital Health'. Which is perfectly fine! That being said, people—all of us—have the power to push for change and progress.

People

The aphorism 'knowledge is power' is an apt one. Because of the Digital and Genomic Revolutions, we are increasingly afforded a wealth of previously-unavailable information about our bodies, our personal disease risk, and what can keep us healthy. The biggest health-related opportunity to ride the Fourth Wave is in the hands of all of us: the knowledge that physical activity is vital to our health and wellbeing. As mentioned, 86% of healthcare costs in the United States result from chronic, mostly preventable diseases. Surprisingly, by simply changing our behavior—particularly as it relates to physical activity, nutrition, sleep, and stress—we have the ability to dramatically reduce overall costs in the healthcare system and, in many cases, what we spend out-of-pocket.

Ride the Wave

Nearly 100 years ago, in a 1926 interview, Nikola Tesla—the legendary futurist and designer of the alternating current (AC) electricity supply system—stated the following: "From the inception of the wireless system, I saw that this new art of applied electricity would be of greater benefit to the human race than any other scientific discovery, for it virtually eliminates distance.

The majority of the ills from which humanity suffers are due to the immense extent of the terrestrial globe and the inability of individuals and nations to come into close contact. Wireless will achieve the closer contact through transmission of intelligence, transport of our bodies, and materials, and conveyance of energy. When wireless is perfectly applied the whole earth will be converted into a huge brain, which in fact it is, all things being particles of a real and rhythmic whole. We shall be able to communicate with one another instantly, irrespective of distance. Not only this, but through television and telephony we shall see and hear one another as perfectly as though we were face to face, despite intervening distances of thousands of miles; and the instruments through which we shall be able to do his will be amazingly simple compared with our present telephone. A man will be able to carry one in his vest pocket."

This brings us back full circle to my professional background that focused on leveraging wireless and digital technologies within the aerospace, medical devices, and mobile phone industries. Adding the Digital Revolution with wireless brought Tesla's vision to reality. And in the same way, the Digital Revolution brought Toffler's Third Wave into being. Now, with the addition of the Genomic Revolution, our biology—our genetic code—is creating the Fourth Wave. Our DNA is digital, and genomics innovators like J. Craig Venter are converting between the two and creating a wealth of opportunities for improving human health. Social media, ubiquitous sensors and sensing systems, and brain-computer interfaces add additional layers of value.

Combined with analytics and artificially intelligent (AI) systems, and we're now at the beginning of the Fourth Wave.

Societal checks and balances and judicious controls—including those performed by public, policymakers, regulators, and market forces—will continue to shape this rapidly accelerating new era of human and technological progress. The emerging Fourth Wave is unevenly distributed, imperfect and, unfortunately, sometimes inequitable. However, as with previous great waves of human progress, the transformation will ultimately result in a net benefit to society.

In a 2011 Wall Street Journal essay, Marc Andreessen—a venture capitalist (VC) and the cofounder of Netscape—famously wrote that "Software will eat the world." Andreessen was correct: Software *has* eaten the world. Every aspect of our lives and every sector of the economy has been affected by and transformed by the Digital Revolution.

Society is transitioning from a digital age-driven sociocultural evolution—the Third Wave—into a new era of human progress driven by the fusion of the Digital and Genomic Revolutions, aka digital health, aka The Fourth Wave. This convergence is comprised of innovations and discoveries—digital technology and genomics—that were previously thought to be separate, even dichotomous, but are in fact both digital. The trajectory of innovation, adoption, and aggregate outcomes produced by these two revolutions is mutually amplified and greater than the sum of its parts.

Over the course of the next five, ten, and twenty years, The Fourth Wave: Digital Health will create profound changes in health, healthcare, living, and society. It will be an exciting ride, with each of us contributing to creating this new era of human progress.

Stay abreast of the latest news relevant to The Fourth Wave: Digital Health by subscribing to Paul Sonnier's newsletter at FourthWaveBook.com or StoryofDigitalHealth.com

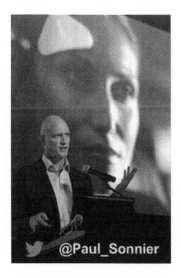

@Paul_Sonnier

Point your iPhone or Android smartphone camera at the QR code and receive a prompt to visit my website